Infecting Ourselves: How Environmental and Social Disruptions Trigger Disease

ANNE E. PLATT

Tonje Vetleseter, *Research Intern*

Jane A. Peterson, *Editor*

WITHDRAW

WORLDWATCH PAPER 129
April 1996

THE WORLDWATCH INSTITUTE is an independent, nonprofit environmental research organization in Washington, D.C. Its mission is to foster a sustainable society in which human needs are met in ways that do not threaten the health of the natural environment or future generations. To this end, the Institute conducts interdisciplinary research on emerging global issues, the results of which are published and disseminated to decision makers and the media.

FINANCIAL SUPPORT is provided by Carolyn Foundation, the Nathan Cummings Foundation, the Geraldine R. Dodge Foundation, the Energy Foundation, The Ford Foundation, the George Gund Foundation, The William and Flora Hewlett Foundation, W. Alton Jones Foundation, John D. and Catherine T. MacArthur Foundation, Andrew W. Mellon Foundation, The Curtis and Edith Munson Foundation, Edward John Noble Foundation, The Pew Charitable Trusts, Lynn R. and Karl E. Prickett Fund, Rockefeller Brothers Fund, Rockefeller Financial Services, Surdna Foundation, Turner Foundation, U.N. Population Fund, Wallace Genetic Foundation, Weeden Foundation, and the Winslow Foundation.

PUBLICATIONS of the Institute include the annual *State of the World*, which is now published in 27 languages; *Vital Signs*, an annual compendium of global trends that are shaping our future; the *Environmental Alert* book series; *World Watch* magazine; and the Worldwatch Papers. For more information on Worldwatch publications, write: Worldwatch Institute, 1776 Massachusetts Ave., NW, Washington, DC 20036; or fax 202-296-7365; or see back pages.

THE WORLDWATCH PAPERS provide in-depth, quantitative and qualitative analysis of the major issues affecting prospects for a sustainable society. The Papers are written by members of the Worldwatch Institute research staff and reviewed by experts in the field. Published in five languages, they have been used as concise and authoritative references by governments, nongovernmental organizations, and educational institutions worldwide. For a partial list of available Papers, see back pages.

DATA from all graphs and tables contained in this Paper are available on 3 1/2" Macintosh or IBM-compatible computer disks. The disks also include data from the *State of the World* series, *Vital Signs*, *Environmental Alert* book series, Worldwatch Papers, and *World Watch* magazine. Each yearly subscription includes a mid-year update, and *Vital Signs* and *State of the World* as they are published. The disk is formatted for Lotus 1-2-3, and can be used with Quattro Pro, Excel, SuperCalc, and many other spreadsheets. To order, see back pages.

Table of Contents

Sections of this paper may be reproduced in magazines and newspapers with written permission from the Worldwatch Institute. For information, call the Director of Communication at (202)452-1999 or Fax: (202)296-7365.

Dedicated to all of the people fighting against AIDS
and other infectious diseases.

ACKNOWLEDGMENTS: Thanks to Marc Lappé, Bennett Lorber, and Robert Shope for their timely and invaluable reviews, as well as to Paul Epstein for his review, input, and encouragement throughout the development of the paper. Thanks to Stephen Morse and Dorothy Preslar for their help. Thanks to my colleagues at Worldwatch: Chris Bright, Chris Flavin, John Young, and Janet Abramovitz for their critical and inspiring reviews. From outlines to bluelines, thanks to my editor, Jane Peterson, for her expertise, patience, and good humor. I owe a debt of gratitude to Denise Byers Thomma, who helped me write a paper and plan a wedding at the same time; Jim Perry, as champion of the media, who pushed me to make this relevant; and Jennifer Seher, for her skills and limitless energy in designing many versions of the paper. Also, thanks to Lori Baldwin, Suzanne Clift, Suzanne Hollander, Laura Malinowski, David Roodman, Aaron Sachs, Payal Sampat, and other Worldwatchers for their help with figures, data and citation checking, and review of particular sections. Thanks to Tonje Vetleseter who contributed thorough research and significant input in the first stages of the paper. Finally, heartfelt thanks to Joe McGinn for standing by me.

ANNE E. PLATT is a Research Associate at the Worldwatch Institute where she focuses on environmental health and fisheries issues. She is coauthor of the Institute's *State of the World 1996* report and contributes regularly to *Vital Signs* and *World Watch* magazine. Previously, she worked at the Environmental Law Institute. In March 1995, Ms. Platt's article on the reemergence of tuberculosis was awarded one of the "Ten Best Censored Stories of 1994," by Sonoma State University's Project Censored.

Introduction

In 1967, the United States Surgeon General, William H. Stewart, announced that the time had come "to close the book on infectious diseases." Proud of their arsenal of medical weaponry and the stunning declines of polio, typhoid, and smallpox, world health officials, like Stewart, pursued nothing short of complete eradication of microbes.[1]

Yet today, less than 30 years after that declaration of victory, infectious diseases are still the leading cause of death in the world, killing more people than cancer and heart disease combined. The organisms that trigger communicable disease continue to evade extensive efforts to bring them under control, and in many places their incidence is again on the rise. Because most health experts have neglected to develop adequate understanding of the life cycles of microbes, the mechanics of infection, or the broader ecology of disease, we have not only failed to break the chain of infection, we have in some instances actually strengthened it. If current trends continue, humanity can soon expect an epidemic of epidemics.[2]

According to official estimates, infectious diseases killed more than 16.5 million people in 1993 worldwide and accounted for one-third of human mortality, though both figures would be significantly higher if accurate data collection were universal. By comparison, the death toll that same year from chronic diseases, such as cancer and heart disease, was 15.6 million. The trends are complex: illness and death from tuberculosis (TB), malaria, dengue fever, and HIV/AIDS are up significantly in the last two decades, but diarrheal diseases, and many childhood diseases, are in decline or under control. While much attention has been focused on recently emerging contagious diseases, most of the big killers are anything but new. Indeed, they have plagued humanity for centuries: Hippocrates described the symptoms of malaria, mumps, diphtheria, tuberculosis, and influenza some 2,300 years ago.[3]

Since 1973, however, at least 30 previously unknown diseases have made their debut on the world stage, including Lyme disease, Legionnaire's disease, and Toxic Shock Syndrome. Moreover, several of the world's most lethal microbes have mounted dangerous counterattacks against antibiotics and other drugs. Diseases such as malaria and tuberculosis have evolved drug-resistant strains that are difficult to control, expensive to treat, and nearly impossible to prevent from spreading. And as people intrude ever more deeply into ecosystems, infections such as salmonella and yellow fever are beginning to cross back and forth between animals and humans. Infectious diseases are also taking a toll on plants.[4]

Invisible to the naked eye, microbes are a formidable foe, not least because they are essential to life. The word microbe—which encompasses bacteria, viruses, and fungi—means *small life* in Greek. Serving as the catalysts for decay and decomposition, microbes process chemicals and transfer material and energy from dead organic material into a form that can be reused by plants and animals.[5]

Many microbes have a mutually productive relationship with their host. Millions of bacteria live in people's intestinal tracts to help the digestive process. And peas and beans host certain bacteria in their roots that convert nitrogen from the atmosphere into a form usable to these plants. Other microbes, however, which are the object of focus here, are pathogenic—that is, they can cause disease.[6]

Bacteria and viruses—which cause most infectious disease—have several traits that help them elude efforts to pin them down. For one thing, they can replicate in a matter of days or less—some active viral infections can produce 1,000 copies in about an hour. In addition, microbes can change their genetic makeup much faster than human cells. Viruses, for instance, are a million times more likely to mutate than human cells. Such traits give these microscopic organisms an evolutionary advantage during periods of massive fluctuation such as the present. This suggests that regaining the uneasy balance that has long existed between microbes and hosts—rather than achieving total victory—must be the objective of public health efforts.[7]

Both the complexity and the diversity of natural ecosystems serve to keep infectious organisms and disease vectors in check.

Both the complexity and the diversity of natural ecosystems serve to keep infectious organisms and disease vectors in check. Disturbing these ecosystems creates new opportunities for microbes to evolve and spread, thereby increasing human vulnerability to infection. Lyme disease, for example, is caused by a bacterium that is carried by ticks. With the decline of wolves and other predatory species that cull herds, deer have multiplied, as have rodents, providing a moveable feast for ticks. First identified in the United States some 20 years ago, Lyme disease now infects 13,000 Americans a year.[8]

Human interference with the natural flow of freshwater systems has also accelerated the spread of infectious disease. Dams and irrigation canals, for instance, often serve as breeding areas for mosquitoes that carry yellow fever and malaria. And water pollution can spark outbreaks of cholera and dysentery.

The planet has become more vulnerable also because it is, in effect, smaller. Distances that were once rarely traversed within the life-span of a microbe are now covered routinely and easily in a day, thanks to expanded air travel, new roads cutting through wilderness areas, and greatly increased trade.

Social changes such as widening poverty, increasing

urbanization, and expanding civil strife have also made humans more vulnerable to infection. Increasing population density and changing lifestyles have contributed to the current pandemic of HIV/AIDS, for example. Although rich countries are also experiencing more frequent outbreaks of contagious disease, the burden is felt most intensely in poor nations.[9]

The environment in which humans evolved and developed their basic defenses against disease was one that remained—despite occasional natural disturbances—basically stable for thousands of years. Then, during the Middle Ages and, later, the Industrial Revolution, enormous population changes led to outbreaks of disease, including the bubonic plague (Black Death), syphilis, and cholera. As the twenty-first century approaches, however, changes of unprecedented magnitude and speed are taking place in the planet's physical and social environment. World population has doubled in the past 40 years. And the number of people living in cities rose from 737 million in 1950 to 2.6 billion in 1995. During the 1980s alone, the world lost 150 million hectares—eight percent—of its tropical forests. The rate at which species are vanishing exceeds natural extinction rates by 100 to 1,000 times. The resulting reduction of biological diversity may cut off or completely eliminate control species that keep microbes in check, as happened with Lyme disease.[10]

Human-induced climate change may soon be another contributor to the spread of infectious disease. Carbon dioxide emissions from fossil fuel burning—nearly 25 billion tons in 1995—have pushed atmospheric concentrations of carbon dioxide to their highest level in 150,000 years, and, with other greenhouse gases, have destabilized the earth's atmosphere. Climate change has the potential to disrupt natural ecosystems, and unleash a variety of microorganisms that spread dangerous diseases.[11]

Finally, overuse and misapplication of antibiotics—the drugs once thought to be the ultimate weapon against infectious disease—have spurred microbes to evolve deadlier

strains of contagion. With some diseases, such as enterococcal infection, just one drug remains to hold the line, and
it is only a matter of time before the bacteria find a way
around that barrier.[12]

The cumulative effects of human interference with
ecosystems allow infections to spread far faster than anyone
has been able to disseminate the means of preventing and
treating them. And as experience with antibiotics has
shown, there is no silver bullet that will stop infectious disease. Our best defenses are simply prevention and informed
action based on awareness of human susceptibility; local,
regional, and global environmental conditions; and
prospects for microbial evolution.

Widespread immunization programs, public education,
safe drinking water, proper sanitation, reliable health services, adequate medical supplies, and other cost-effective
public health measures—and reducing ecological disruptions—can protect millions of people from illness and death.
On the other hand, letting down our guard and short-
changing prevention can have serious consequences, as the
explosion of HIV/AIDS has shown.[13]

Many of these strategies are already being implemented,
but money is desperately needed to expand public health
efforts. Prevention is far less expensive than treatment.
Health economists estimate that every U.S. dollar spent on
the polio vaccine saves $6. Every dollar spent for measles,
mumps, and rubella vaccine saves $21; and every dollar
spent for diphtheria, tetanus, and pertussis vaccine saves
$29. Based on current projections for the eradication of
polio, the World Health Organization (WHO) predicts an
annual global savings of $3 billion by the year 2000.[14]

More selective and frugal use of antibiotics would go a
long way toward slowing the spread of drug resistance.
Recently, for instance, Hungary reduced the number of penicillin-resistant cases of pneumonia by 20 percent in just
three years by encouraging doctors to limit their use of
antibiotics.[15]

WHO, the United Nations Children's Fund (UNICEF),

and other groups have strengthened infectious disease detection and screening networks. Clearly, more of this must be done. It is crucial that governments work together to establish environmental monitoring systems that track weather patterns, map out vector species, predict conditions conducive to outbreaks, and warn people at risk. This type of surveillance also makes it easier and cheaper to target intervention to those who need it most.[16]

With another 3 to 5 billion people likely to be added to the world's population by 2050, and human-induced climate change already being detected by scientists, the current crisis of infectious disease is almost certain to deepen. This tragedy is unnecessary, according to the director-general of the World Health Organization, because the medical knowledge and resources exist to treat and control many infectious diseases. By emphasizing prevention, and modifying our current development policies—from high rates of energy and resource consumption to disruptive land use practices and destabilizing population trends—we can keep infections from taking hold in the first place.[17]

The Burden and Challenge of Infectious Disease

Many infectious diseases are preventable or easily treated, so the fact that they continue to impose a great burden is largely a reflection of policy choices. The resurgence of some diseases, for example, has more to do with deterioration of public health services than with lack of knowledge. Because of cutbacks, community health efforts promoting attention to water supply, immunization, hygiene, preventive medicine, and education have fallen off. This is dangerous timing, especially in view of the fact that many infectious diseases now have antibiotic-resistant strains that may cause higher death counts in the future.[18]

The top five infectious killers of humans are acute respiratory infections such as pneumonia (4.1 million deaths), diarrheal diseases (3 million), tuberculosis (2.7 million), malaria (2 million), and measles (1.2 million). (See Table 1.) More than 98 percent of deaths from communicable diseases (16.3 million) occur in developing countries. Worldwide, infectious diseases account for 32 percent of deaths from all causes but in developing countries they cause 42 percent of total deaths. In industrial countries, by contrast, microbes are responsible for only 1.2 percent of deaths (200,000).[19]

While suffering and loss caused by contagious diseases are concentrated in developing countries, industrial countries carry a growing share of the problem. In the United States, for example, where public attention shifted to cancer and heart disease some time ago, deaths from infectious diseases jumped 58 percent between 1980 and 1992, from 41 to 65 deaths per 100,000. Much of the increase came from a rise in HIV/AIDS and respiratory infections, such as pneumonia. In 1994, infectious diseases were the underlying cause of death in 8 percent of nearly 2.2 million U.S. fatalities, ranking third as the leading cause of death after heart disease and malignant neoplasms (cancers).[20]

In addition to killing millions of people worldwide, infections cause chronic and debilitating illness for millions more, particularly in developing countries. For example, an estimated 1.8 billion episodes of diarrheal disease occurred in 1993, primarily in Sub-Saharan Africa. Acute respiratory infections such as bronchitis and influenza cause millions of cases but few deaths, in comparison. In 1993, one in ten people on earth—some 570 million people living in Africa, Asia, and Latin America—were infected with tropical diseases such as malaria, African trypanosomiasis (sleeping sickness), onchocerciasis (river blindness), and schistosomiasis (bilharziasis). (See Table 1.) In addition, there are more than a hundred other obscure infectious diseases carried by water, soil, food, and vectors.[21]

Some diseases, like measles and smallpox, can be easily eradicated because they demonstrate fairly predictable life

Disease				Type / Transmission	Symptoms
AIDS (Acquired Immunodeficiency Syndrome)	(AIDS) 0.6 (HIV) 4.0	0.7	>	Virus, HIV, types 1 & 2 sexual contact	Autoimmune dysfunction progresses from asymptomatic to lethal; any organ system can be targeted. Initially: fever, weight loss, diarrhea, fatigue, cough, skin lesions, lympha-denopathy; then, opportunistic infections and cancers are common, including TB
Whooping cough (pertussis)	4.3	0.4	<	Bacterium, airborne	Hacking cough, infection of respiratory tract, paroxysmal cough going from high to low pitch; can cause pneumonia & brain damage, even death
Meningitis	1.2*	0.2	>	Bacterium & virus, airborne	Inflammation of meninges of brain & spinal cord
Schistosomiasis	200.0*	0.2	>	Protozoan, snail-borne	Cirrhosis of liver, & anemia
Leishmaniasis	13.0	0.2	>	Protozoan, sandfly	Skin lesions, inflammation & crusting, skin ulcers, tissue destruction in nose & mouth

Sources: See endnote 19.
* Prevalence

TABLE 1

Characteristics of Major Infectious Diseases, 1993 estimates, by Death Counts

Disease	Incidence (millions)	Deaths (millions)	Trends	Vector	Symptoms
Acute Respiratory infections	248.0	4.1	>	Bacterium & virus, airborne	Cold, sore throat, influenza, pneumonia, & bronchitis
Diarrheal diseases	1,800.0	3.0	<	Bacterium & virus, water & food-borne	Frequent liquid stools, sometimes bloody
Tuberculosis	8.8	2.7	>	Bacterium, airborne	Severe coughing, sometimes with blood, chest pain, exhaustion, weight loss, & night sweats
Malaria	400.0*	2.0	>	Protozoan, mosquito-borne	Fever, headache, nausea, vomiting, diarrhea, myalgias, malaise, enlarged spleen, liver, renal & respiratory failure, shock, pulmonary & cerebral endema
Measles	45.0	1.2	<	Virus, airborne	Rash & fever, encephalitis in rare cases
Hepatitis B	4.2	1.0	>	Virus, sexual contact	Anorexia, abdominal pain, sometimes rash, jaundice, cirrhosis of liver (chronic infection)

cycles and symptoms, and it is possible to induce immunity to those particular symptoms. More often, however, infections are complex and difficult to control, producing symptoms that vary depending on stages in the life cycle of the microbe and the health of the victim. The malaria protozoan, for instance, has different susceptibilities to antimicrobial drugs at different points in its transmission cycle: in various stages of developing from egg to parasite, in its vector, or in human blood. Malaria is especially difficult to track also because it is actually four diseases caused by *Plasmodium* protozoa that are carried by 60 different *Anopheles* species of mosquitoes. The biology and the breeding behavior of these species vary greatly, so control measures for one species may not work against another.[22]

Despite the formidable problems infectious diseases present, considerable progress in the fight against them has been made during this century. For example, smallpox—a highly infectious virus that is spread by respiration or touch, and can disfigure, blind, and even kill its victim—was declared officially eradicated in 1979. Mounting a concentrated campaign, doctors and health workers vaccinated more than 250 million people against smallpox in countries still besieged by this disease and rid the planet of it in one final heroic effort. And measles has nearly vanished from the industrialized world. In 1994, Finland became the first country to declare itself free of homegrown cases of this fever- and rash-causing illness, which killed more than 1.2 million people worldwide in 1993. In Latin America, the incidence of measles plummeted from 125 per 100,000 in 1963 to under 16 per 100,000 in 1992 due to immunizations.[23]

Polio, a crippling viral disease, also appears to be on the way out; it has already been eliminated in 145 countries reporting to UNICEF's Expanded Program on Immunization (EPI). Worldwide, new cases plunged 80 percent between 1988 and 1994, from 35,000 to 6,000. Europe, North and South America, the South Pacific, and southern and northern Africa reported no indigenous cases of polio in 1994.[24]

Despite the proven benefits of immunization against polio, measles, and other infectious diseases, however, many people are still not immunized. Inexpensive treatments are not distributed widely, and basic infrastructure and administrative problems as well as a lack of money, supplies, personnel, and knowledge hamper further improvements in prevention and treatment.[25]

Another critical obstacle to further progress is the dearth of basic information that is crucial to measuring the impact of infectious disease. Underreporting and misdiagnosis are serious problems in many areas of the world—some diseases were not identified until recently, diagnostic capabilities and surveillance systems do not exist everywhere, and some infectious diseases are simply never recorded. Thus actual incidence may often be many times higher than what is reported. Where no real surveillance occurs, passive and delayed reporting to a central health authority is the norm, and often there is confusion concerning disease identification.[26]

In the United States, deaths from infectious diseases jumped 58 percent between 1980 and 1992.

The Nigerian Health Ministry, for example, reported that the 1987 yellow fever epidemic in Oyo State resulted in 883 cases and 477 deaths. Four years later, however, researchers examined epidemiological information and changed the estimate to 116,000 cases and 24,000 deaths. Based on these data, the 11,000 cases of yellow fever reported for all of Africa between 1986 and 1990 may have represented as many as 1.4 million cases. Similarly, Vietnam confirmed more than 350,000 cases of malaria in 1990, but the actual number was more likely on the order of 1.5 million.[27]

The World Health Organization has 190 member states, of which only 60 routinely report data. Forty-seven of these 60 are developed countries, which have the best records but the least number of cases. Global data are, therefore, inherently skewed toward contagious disease in developed countries, where cases are limited and many infections do not occur at all. Some of the countries in Asia and the Americas that keep track of infectious disease have good historical (pre-1980) series. Sub-Saharan Africa countries, for the most part, have little to no historical data, and assessments of long-term trends in infectious diseases are rare. The quality of recent data from most developing countries is inconsistent, a problem that severely limits the ability to maintain effective control programs.[28]

Disease reporting and data collection are often neglected because of money shortages. In situations where health clinics must choose between actual care and data collection, it seems irrational to spend time and resources to count the sick and dying—the money could be better used trying to help them. And yet, even rough estimates of incidence (new cases) and mortality help health officials to allocate resources better and to respond to growing needs for care and research.[29]

Another aspect of this data problem relates to *how* infectious diseases are classified and reported. Generally, they are classified by the target organ in the body, on a disease-by-disease basis, rather than by their communicable or non-communicable nature. For example, otitis media, or middle ear infection, is categorized as an ear disease, not as an infectious disease. Diseases officially classified as infectious represent only the "tip of the iceberg" of disorders caused by infectious agents.[30]

In 1995, researchers from the U. S. Centers for Disease Control and Prevention (CDC) found that codes were listed under infectious diseases or consequences of infection. But less than half of deaths "directly attributable to infectious diseases are labeled explicitly as infectious" in the International Classification of Diseases (ICD), according to a recent study published in the *Journal of the American Medical Association*. To be more accurate, one must analyze each particular disease and determine if it is caused by an infection or results in infectious illness.[31]

Despite problems of classification and counting, the sets

of time-series data (collected over periods of time) available from individual countries and WHO demonstrate clear trends. Until recently, many diseases—such as diphtheria, sleeping sickness, malaria, and tuberculosis—were thought to have been well under control. Yet several infectious diseases have reemerged, or have appeared in human populations for the first time.

Attempts to alter the natural balance of microbe and host can actually lead to more disease.

An epidemic of diphtheria—a flu-like disease that kills 5-10 percent of its victims—originally began in 1990 in Russia and has since spread throughout the former Soviet Union. The incidence of diphtheria in the newly independent states shot up from 839 cases in 1989 to 47,802 in 1994, with three-fourths of this childhood illness striking people over the age of 15. (See Figure 1.) Immunization with the DPT vaccine (for diphtheria, pertussis, tetanus) had virtually stopped by the late 1980s, when the country was undergoing social and political upheaval. As a result, a large percentage of the population lost access to medical care and became susceptible to diphtheria. Similarly, there has been a rise in cases of whooping cough (pertussis).[32]

Cases of African sleeping sickness reported to the Vanga Health Zone in Zaire have risen 10-fold since 1990. And, there are now believed to be more than 1 million unreported cases in rural villages of central African countries such as Angola and Zaire, according to Felix Kuzoe, the WHO Coordinator for Research on African Trypanosomiasis. This disease, which is carried by the tsetse fly, is caused by trypanosomes—microscopic pathogens that infect blood, lymph glands, and eventually the brain. While sleeping sickness is invariably fatal without treatment, early intervention leads to cure in 90 percent of cases.[33]

Although malaria was thought to be under control in the 1960s, drug-resistant strains of the *Plasmodium* protozoan have led to its resurgence. Malaria cases officially reported to WHO's Africa regional office jumped from 3 million to 23 million between 1983 and 1988. (Reporting in that region has virtually stopped since 1990, primarily because of civil disorder.) Cases in the Americas went from 830,000 in 1983 to 1.1 million in 1992; cases in Southeast Asia also increased by about 300,000—to more than 3 million—during the same time period. Worldwide, cases of malaria reported outside of Africa increased from less than 1 million cases reported between 1960 and 1965, to 5.5 million per year in the late 1980s. A major epidemic occurred in India between 1974 and 1978, with more than 6 million cases reported there alone. Multi-drug-resistant strains of malaria now exist in Southeast Asia; if they spread to Africa it would be "a disaster of immense proportions." In the next decade, the world could easily face a major epidemic wherein a new strain of malaria emerges for which there is no effective drug.[34]

Data for tuberculosis, also known as consumption, demonstrate a dramatic resurgence of this disease as well. In absolute numbers, cases rose from 2.95 million in 1985 to 3.8 million in 1989. Just four years later, an estimated 8.8 million people contracted tuberculosis, more than double the number in 1989. An estimated 2.7 million people died from this severe pulmonary infection in 1993, more than became ill from it eight years earlier.[35]

The recent resurgence of TB needs to be seen in historical context to be appreciated. In 1900, this wasting disease killed 200 Americans for every 100,000 infected, primarily in cities. As public health measures improved, the number of deaths fell to 60 per 100,000 by 1940 in the United States. In developed countries the number of cases remained low, but the number in developing countries climbed. Worldwide, rates of tuberculosis have turned upward, from 61.8 per 100,000 people in 1984-1986, to 74.6 per 100,000 in 1989-91, with the largest increase reported in Southeast Asia (from 115 to 146 per 100,000).[36]

During the 1990s, at least 30 million people are expected to die from tuberculosis as the number of cases compli-

FIGURE 1

Epidemic of Diphtheria in Newly Independent States of the former Soviet Union, 1965–1994

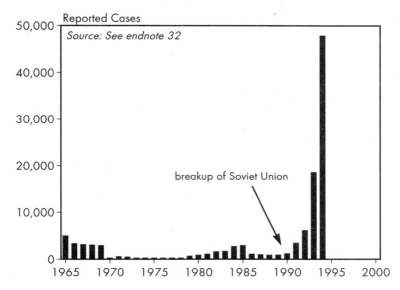

cated by drug-resistant strains and co-infection with HIV rises. In developing countries, where most deaths from TB occur, HIV is spreading quickly, largely because of inadequate health services and poor surveillance. Soon, TB may again become the world's leading killer disease, much as it was in the early 1900s.[37]

But tuberculosis, malaria, and diphtheria are just part of a larger pattern that involves many diseases and increasing risks to hundreds of millions of people. The data demonstrate that human interference with, and attempts to alter, the natural balance of microbe and host can actually lead to more disease.

Outbreaks of infectious disease tend to be clustered in certain areas, depending on local weather and climate, susceptibility of the population, and existing health infrastructure. Also, human population size and density are key variables in determining outbreaks. Together, these factors influence the rate of microbial introduction, the chances of microbes becoming established, the rate of their spread, the evolution of their virulence, and the capacity of human society to defend itself against them.[38]

Cases of drug-resistant pneumonia, for example, are found primarily in industrial countries, where antibiotics are widely overused. And some 90 percent of malaria deaths occur in Sub-Saharan Africa, where tropical conditions are hospitable to the *Anopheles* mosquitoes that transmit this disease. Similarly, much of the suffering from AIDS has been concentrated in Africa because of lack of health care and in Asia because of population density, although Europe and the Americas are hardly immune to this killer. Nearly two-thirds of the world's 13 to 14 million cases of HIV are found in Africa; however, in 1995, for the first time, more people are believed to have contracted HIV in Asia than anywhere else. Worldwide, 1.8 million people died from HIV/AIDS—more than from measles and nearly as many as malaria—up from about 1 million in 1994.[39]

The basic characteristics of microbial life—high rates of replication and mutation, and an ability to adapt to almost any type of external conditions—underlie the broader ecology of communicable disease. They are what makes an infectious disease infectious, capable of being spread to others. In contrast to "opportunistic" microbes, hosts—human beings, plants, and animals—have larger bodies, reproduce later in life, and generate small broods. In a stable environment, hosts are superior competitors and keep opportunistic species, such as microbes, in check. Infections can be best understood as a struggle for survival between host and microbe.[40]

To take hold in a population and then to spread and persist, a microbe needs a certain number of susceptible hosts— a threshold level or critical community size that is large enough to continue the cycle of infection uninterrupted. When a critical percentage of the hosts exposed have become immune, the epidemic stops. Measles epidemics, for example, require at least 500,000 people to provide the required susceptible population of 7,000. Rubella, typhoid, and dysentery emerged and increased as cities grew in the Middle Ages because these infections need populations of 100,000 to 500,000 in order to be transmitted.[41]

Obviously, it is impossible to prevent people from living in crowded areas, but understanding a microbe's need for a certain number of susceptible hosts can help authorities to predict where an outbreak might occur and then take action to stop it from spreading like wildfire.[42]

Most microbes coexist peacefully with their hosts. But this is an uneasy balance that can be upset in a number of ways. Disruptions in a host's immune system, in the environment at large, or within the microbe can activate a latent (harmless) infection and cause disease to emerge or reemerge. And these disruptions intersect in complicated ways. (See Table 2.)[43]

The basic characteristics of microbial life— an ability to adapt to almost any type of external conditions— underlie the broader ecology of communicable disease.

For many microbes, survival is a difficult balancing act. Lest its own life be cut short, a pathogen cannot be so lethal that it kills its host before spreading to a new victim. On the other hand, it must be strong enough to replicate within its host and have a fairly good chance of being transmitted. Interestingly, some microbes survive in humans and other hosts without causing illness; in fact, the more successful ones often do not harm their reservoir host (where they complete their life cycle and development). For the purposes of spreading infection, an immune host (as distinct from a reservoir host) is not much different from a dead one; both serve as a dead end for pathogens.[44]

The particular requirements of microbes mean that it is not necessary to vaccinate absolutely everyone to build immunity in a host population; only the majority of the

TABLE 2

Causes of Infectious Disease Emergence, Representative Disease Examples

Cause of Emergence	Infectious Disease
Changing Environmental Conditions	
Deforestation	Malaria, hemorrhagic fevers, rabies, Lyme disease
Agriculture and irrigation	Argentine hemorrhagic fever, Japanese encephalitis, Bolivian hemorrhagic fever, schistosomiasis, influenza (pandemic)
Dam building, road building	Schistosomiasis, malaria, Rift Valley fever
Poor sanitation and hygiene	Diarrheal diseases, malaria, schistosomiasis, lymphatic filariasis, onchocerciasis (River blindness), dengue, yellow fever, cholera, dracunculiasis (Guinea worm disease), Japanese encephalitis, *Salmonella*, *Escherichia coli* O157:H7 (Hemolytic uremic syndrome), cryptosporidiosis, giardia
Climate change	Hanta virus, plague, malaria, schistosomiasis, other vector-borne diseases
Demographic Changes	
Urbanization	Yellow fever, malaria, dengue, acute respiratory illnesses, plague, cholera
Increased trade, travel, and migration	Cholera, yellow fever, influenza, dengue and dengue hemorrhagic fever, pneumonia, HIV/AIDS, influenza
Deteriorating Social Conditions	
Breakdown in public health services	Measles, diphtheria, pertussis, tuberculosis, cholera, influenza, HIV/AIDS, and other sexually transmitted diseases (STDs)

War and civil disorder	Malaria, cholera, diphtheria, waterborne diseases
Increased sexual activity	Hepatitis B and C, HIV/AIDS, STDs
Intravenous drug use	HIV/AIDS
Overuse of antibiotics	Antibiotic-resistant strains of malaria, tuberculosis, staphylocci, pneumococci, enterococci, gonorrhea, and others
Other	
Air-conditioning systems	Legionnaire's disease
Ultra-absorbent tampons	Toxic Shock Syndrome
Unknown	*Streptococcus* Group A (necrotizing fasciitis), Ebola

Source: See endnote 43

group needs to be immune. Theoretically, it is only necessary to bring the remaining susceptible population down below the critical threshold level. The threshold level of smallpox, for instance, is about 80 percent of most populations. Mass vaccination offers the easiest, and most reliable, method to prevent some infectious diseases such as measles and tetanus. Other diseases such as malaria, of course, require a more sophisticated control strategy, especially in view of the fact that humans and microbes are evolving at the same time and in response to one another.[45]

How Social Conditions Speed Up Microbial Traffic

Before Christopher Columbus arrived in the New World at the end of the fifteenth century, an estimated 100 million people lived in the Americas. But foreign pathogens brought by European explorers decimated the aboriginal American peoples. The population of Mexico, for instance, plunged from 20 million to 3 million between 1518 and 1568, then to 1.5 million over the next 50 years, mainly as a result of successive smallpox, measles, and typhus (fever and rash) epidemics.[46]

The movement of people, plants, animals, and goods— known as biological mixing—serves to increase exposure to disease. Any person, plant, or animal that moves can potentially carry a microbe or organism that will be foreign at its destination.   Dr. Stephen Morse, a virologist at Rockefeller University, coined the phrase "viral traffic" to describe the transfer of viruses to new areas, or species. The same idea applies to bacteria and other microorganisms.   Some human-induced conditions serve as a green light for microbial mixing, while others slow or completely halt the flow of traffic, essentially acting as red lights.   As Morse says, "inevitably viral traffic is enhanced by *human* traffic."[47]

Influenza is a classic example of a disease that spreads rapidly. The great influenza pandemic of this century, for instance, broke out in 1918, and within four months it had spread all over the world, carried home by soldiers returning from World War I. Only Iceland and Samoa were spared, and that was before modern air travel. Malnutrition, societal disruption, and under-equipped hospitals after the war boosted the chances of this highly contagious infection spreading. The pandemic killed 20 million people worldwide—more than twice as many as World War I itself.[48]

The world's pandemic strains of influenza are thought to originate in China's integrated duck, pig, and chicken farms. Every year, strains sampled from these settings are analyzed to produce vaccines that are distributed worldwide for the flu season.   Medical authorities encourage people to be immunized against recombined strains of influenza to prevent outbreaks.   Despite these precautions, flu outbreaks cost the United States $5 billion each year in medical expenses.[49]

Where infectious disease is concerned, geographically

isolated populations no longer exist. With 1 million people daily crossing international borders by air, an infectious pathogen, such as influenza, can easily travel around the world in a matter of hours. The likelihood of an isolated case causing a serious medical problem is rather small, but rapidly increasing rates of travel boost the chances that such cases will become more frequent and have long-lasting effects on susceptible populations. The dengue 3 strain, for instance, which recently arrived in Central America and is spreading rapidly throughout the region, is a Sri Lankan/South Indian strain.[50]

In the 1980s, DHF emerged throughout Latin America, where it increased 60-fold between 1989 and 1994.

Simply moving the microbes and vectors to new places is not enough to start an epidemic. There must be large enough populations of hosts and victims to ensure the chain of infection. And the social, ecological, and climatological conditions must be conducive to the spread of disease. Dengue, for instance, is carried by the female *Aedes aegypti* mosquito, which also transmits yellow fever. The mosquitoes thrive in urban areas, living and breeding in small containers of water such as flower pots, tires, birdbaths, gutters, barrels, and even plastic covers. They are hardy urban survivors and can be found in nearly every major city in the tropics. Each year, up to 100 million people are infected with dengue fever; nearly half of the world's population is at risk of infection.[51]

Cases of dengue—also known as breakbone fever because of the kind of pain it causes—have been on the rise in Latin America since the 1980s at a time of increasing urbanization and cutbacks in mosquito control programs. As the mosquito population has increased, so have cases of dengue fever and dengue hemorrhagic fever.[52]

Meanwhile, another successful vector of dengue, *Ae. albopictus*—better known as the Asian tiger mosquito—

established itself in the southeastern United States, extending its range southward into Latin America and northward toward Chicago and Washington, D.C. Originally introduced to Texas in a 1985 shipment of used tires from Asia, the Asian tiger mosquito is a more vicious biter and can survive cold winters better than its tropical cousin. In the past 10 years, cases of dengue have been reported only in isolated outbreaks in several U.S. cities, including Houston, but officials are concerned that the fever could become established in North America. In 1994, roughly 20,000 people in Puerto Rico were infected with this disease.[53]

One of the difficulties of combatting dengue is that there are several types, and being infected with one does not give a person permanent immunity to the others. Sequential infections of the different viruses can trigger dengue hemorrhagic fever (DHF), characterized by internal bleeding, and can lead to dengue shock syndrome (DSS), a more severe form of dengue hemorrhagic fever. The exact progression from dengue fever to DHF and DSS is not known.[54]

DHF first appeared in Manila in 1953 and spread quickly through Southeast Asia in the 1960s. In the 1980s, DHF emerged in Brazil, Cuba, and Venezuela and eventually moved throughout Latin America, where it increased 60-fold between 1989 and 1994. As the rapid spread of dengue fever shows, biological mixing, population growth, urbanization, environmental change, travel, and poverty often serve as microbial green lights, in effect telling microbes to proceed. Understanding these traffic signals makes it easier to control the traffic.[55]

At the same time that world population has doubled, in the last 40 years, the world's most vulnerable sub-populations—those living in urban areas, and those struck by poverty, malnutrition, and, increasingly, AIDS—have increased dramatically. Today, nearly 45 percent of the world's population (2.6 billion people) live in an urban area, and by 2025, an estimated 60 percent (4 billion people) will be city-dwellers. As people migrate from rural to urban areas, many will live in peri-urban areas, slums, and squatter settlements, creating rich breeding grounds for infectious disease. A 1983 study found that mortality rates from tuberculosis were three times higher in the slums of Buenos Aires than in the rest of the city itself. Sickness and deaths from diarrheal diseases, respiratory infections, and childhood infections are consistently higher in slums and poor areas of cities like Durban, Guatemala City, Seoul, and Saõ Paulo, than in the wealthier sections of these cities.[56]

The poor are more vulnerable to infectious disease, partly because they are less able to afford food and shelter, let alone medical care or treatment. Accordingly, the director-general of the World Health Organization, Dr. Hiroshi Nakajima, calls poverty "the world's deadliest disease...the main reason why babies are not vaccinated, why clean water and sanitation are not provided, and why curative drugs are unavailable." Malnutrition resulting from poverty, and lack of clean water are leading causes of diarrheal diseases among children. Malnutrition weakens the body's immune system, making it less able to fight infection.[57]

Where conditions conducive to infection occur, the microbial traffic lights can be identified and certain patterns of infection can be expected. Some infectious diseases— such as tuberculosis, influenza, measles, diphtheria, and HIV/AIDS—are transmitted person to person and directly reflect disrupted social conditions. Other diseases—such as malaria, dengue, and the plague—are more directly related to environmental *and* social changes. Lifestyle choices and individual behavior also increase the chances of some diseases spreading, for example sexually transmitted diseases like herpes, syphilis, and HIV/AIDS. Sometimes, opportunistic infections take advantage of each other, as co-infection of HIV/AIDS and TB shows.[58] (See Table 2.)

Probably the most dramatic example of an emerging infectious disease is HIV/AIDS, whose spread was aided by the paving of the Kinshasa Highway from Point-Noire, Zaire, to Mombasa, Kenya, in the 1970s. Although the origin of the AIDS virus, HIV, is not known, its initial eruption among humans was most likely exacerbated by human migration and behavior.[59]

Every year, an average of 4 million people contract HIV, more than the total number infected between 1975 and 1985. By 1994, more than 25 million people worldwide were infected with HIV, and between 5 and 9 million had developed full-blown AIDS. (See Figure 2.) Most cases are in Africa, but WHO experts agree that the pandemic has just begun in South Asia. India's National AIDS Control Organization of the Health Ministry estimates that the 1.5 million HIV infections reported in 1995 in India alone will mushroom into more than 5 million by the year 2000. By 2010, nearly 30 million Indians will be HIV-positive, if current trends continue—more than the total number of HIV-infected people worldwide in 1994.[60]

The spread of HIV has proved particularly difficult to control because it takes about 10 years for the infection to develop into a full-blown case of AIDS. Thus, infected patients can transmit HIV even though they may show no signs of disease, and patients often spread the infection unknowingly to others.[61]

HIV is transmitted through sexual intercourse or exposure to HIV-infected blood, semen, or organs; or from an infected woman to her fetus or infant. In Africa and Asia, HIV/AIDS has spread primarily through heterosexual contact. Prostitutes and commercial sex workers in Southeast Asia were among the first in that region to contract AIDS. In China, nearly half of all people with HIV live in Yunnan province, in the southern part of the country, bordering Myanmar, Laos, and Vietnam. This area is known for its heavy drug trade and, increasingly, for AIDS.[62]

Despite their small relative share of cases—5 percent—industrial countries are not immune to AIDS's deadly call. AIDS became the number one slayer of American adults ages 25 to 44 in 1992. While the initial epidemic in the United States was reported among homosexual populations, more recently, transmission rates have increased through heterosexual contact. In 1994, about 75 percent of HIV infections

FIGURE 2

Global HIV/AIDS Infections, Cumulative, 1980–1995

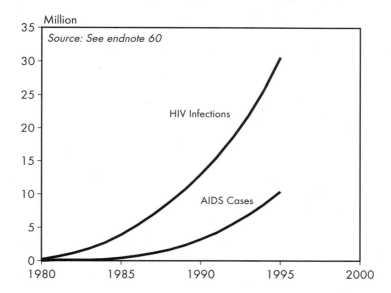

occurred among intravenous drug users and addicts.[63]

The impact this pandemic is having on demographic trends is astonishing: in the United States, one in three African-American men, one in five African-American women, and one in twenty white men will develop AIDS during their lifetime if current trends continue. These data speak to enormous changes in the demographic picture, not only in the United States, but worldwide as well. In Uganda, for instance, life expectancy already plummeted from 52 to 42 years between 1980 and 1994, because of AIDS. In Thailand, known for its rapid economic growth, life expectancy is predicted to drop by nearly half, from 69 years in 1994 to 40 years by 2010, largely because of AIDS.[64]

From the beginning of the pandemic, HIV has cut across all demographic groups. In Zimbabwe, half of the country's soldiers are HIV-infected, as well as a large share of its well-educated, highly skilled working adults. Similarly, in Thailand, the disease has taken a high toll among the coun-

try's elite—those who can afford recreational drugs, prostitutes, and expensive travel. In other countries, such as
India, Cambodia, Uganda, and inner-city areas of the United
States, AIDS is a leading killer of migrant workers, the under-
educated, and the poor.[65]

Because of this enormous human toll, AIDS is more than
simply a health issue: it is a development issue, an economic issue, and a human rights issue. Most victims are afflict-
ed in the prime of their working years, and unable to support their families or to work productively. In Zimbabwe,
one out of four adults is now infected with HIV. In 1993, the
AIDS pandemic cost the world an estimated US$11 billion in
direct health care costs. A research report by DRI/McGraw
Hill estimates that the AIDS pandemic will cost Asian countries alone $52 billion by the end of the century, primarily
in lost productivity.[66]

In addition to morbidity and mortality, AIDS exacts a
high emotional and physical price from family members
who are spared the illness. It greatly increases their stress
and means that time spent on learning and other productive
work is sacrificed for labor and care-giving. Development
officials predict that the disease will severely impact
advances made in reducing infant mortality rates and primary education in the near future. In Tanzania, AIDS death
rates among children may cut enrollment in school by an
average 20 percent. UNICEF estimates that by 1999, more
than 5 million African children will have lost their mothers
to AIDS. Orphaned by this disease, many children themselves will succumb to it as well, or die of neglect.[67]

Just recognizing that the problem of AIDS exists has
been a tough challenge in developing and developed countries alike. Public education about this and other sexually
transmitted diseases is often silenced because it conflicts
with religious and cultural beliefs about gender roles and
sexuality. But it has become difficult to ignore a disease that
even Buddhist monks—who seem so isolated from the rav-
ages of a sexually transmitted epidemic—now contract in
Thailand. Slowly, countries are beginning to admit and con-

front one of the most terrible plagues humanity has ever known.[68]

Because so much of the world is now affected by AIDS, development officials, public health workers, and political leaders have begun to recognize a need to address this public health crisis for economic and social reasons. Distribution of condoms, health screening, HIV testing, education, and prevention strategies aimed at vulnerable populations have helped to bring infection rates down in some areas. In Cambodia, the National AIDS Committee has worked to raise understanding, promote safer sex, and remove misconceptions that can lead to discrimination. In Harare, Zimbabwe, sexually transmitted disease rates fell 63 percent following condom promotion. These diseases greatly increase vulnerability to HIV/AIDS.[69]

How Environmental Disturbances Stimulate Microbes

From the days of Hippocrates until a little over a century ago, some doctors believed that sudden outbreaks of illness were caused by miasma (noxious emanation) emerging from rotting corpses in the earth. When miasma encountered weakened hosts, disease resulted. This theory dominated scientific thinking through the mid-nineteenth century. Most medical scientists left humans out of the picture of risks and underlying causes of disease, until 1880, when the development of the microscope enabled Robert Koch to discover bacteria, specifically, tubercle bacilli.[70]

Although the miasmatic theory of disease may seem mystical, it does carry a grain of truth: that many infectious diseases are related to, and even caused by, something in the environment. All ecological disruptions—such as fire, flood, deforestation, earthquake, and land use changes—tip the balance between people and microbes in favor of microbes. Humans play a larger role in the spread of diseases than they realize through ecological disruption over which they have some control: development projects, large-scale resource extraction activities, and land use changes resulting from logging, agriculture, migration, and urbanization.[71]

Even though each infectious disease has its own distinct characteristics—its own method of transmission, symptoms, and target population—all take advantage of general environmental patterns that upset the normal coexistence between microbes and humans. (See Table 2.) So, as we inflict damage on our environment, we become more vulnerable to opportunistic species, such as pathogenic microbes. While it is unnecessary to halt development, people can be more intelligent about the way they change the face of the earth.

In most examples of ecological change, microbes are circulating in natural hosts. Human activities such as agriculture and logging can amplify transmission of those microbes. Then, when susceptible human hosts move into these altered landscapes disease is more likely to take hold and spark an outbreak.[72]

Specialists refer to "manmade malaria" to describe the routine phenomenon of the disease flaring up near irrigation projects, dams, construction sites, standing water, and poorly drained areas where malaria is already present during seasons when conditions are right for mosquitoes. Such outbreaks are common throughout the tropical areas of Asia, Africa, and the Americas.[73]

For instance, after the Indira Gandhi Canal was built in the state of Rajasthan in 1958, to irrigate desert-like areas of India, farmers switched from cultivating traditional crops of jowar and bajra to more commercially profitable wheat and cotton, which require large amounts of water. Many people came to the area in search of work. The main canal—445 kilometers long—turned out to be an ideal breeding site for mosquitoes during the monsoon season. Instead of high crop productivity and prosperity, the heavy rains brought the farmers rapidly spreading cerebral malaria, which untreated can quickly kill by causing the brain to hemorrhage. Malaria (and now dengue fever) and waterborne diseases are common during India's monsoon season, but the canals carried the epidemic to a much larger area, exposing workers and farmers.[74]

A different project in the region—India's Sardar Sarovar Dam—has sparked epidemics as well. Here, "the ignition wire of construction-related stagnant water, and the gunpowder of immigrant labor, [create] an explosion of malaria," reported a World Bank-commissioned independent review of the project.[75]

Even without irrigation, converting land to agricultural use can increase exposure to new diseases. For centuries, the fertile temperate

All ecological disruptions tip the balance between people and microbes in favor of microbes.

pampas area of Argentina supported cattle, weeds, grasses, and wild fauna. Maize and alfalfa production was introduced to the northwestern provinces of the country during the 1920s, and by the 1940s herbicides were being heavily applied to control the native grasses and weeds. Grasses that could withstand the herbicides and grow in the shade under maize stalks began to take over, and a once-rare rodent—the field mouse, *Calomys musculinus*—became dominant. This rodent had long lived in the pampas, but in small numbers. Feeding on the seeds of these newly dominant plants, however, the field mouse thrived and proliferated in maize and alfalfa fields. Unfortunately, it is the vector and natural reservoir of Junín virus, which causes Argentine hemorrhagic fever. And, when the tall grasses disappeared, so did the mouse's natural predators.[76]

With growing populations of mice, farmers became exposed to the Junín virus. Since its discovery in 1958, more than 20,000 Argentineans have been infected. Nearly one-third of these people died from Argentine hemorrhagic fever. Its symptoms include high fever, headache, low blood pressure, vomiting, dehydration, and eventual internal hemorrhaging that causes the body to go into shock and

drown in its own blood.   Modern agricultural equipment
has also spread the disease: combine harvesters occasionally
run over a rodent and create a spray of infective aerosol.
Most of the time, however, rodent droppings are the cul-
prit.[77]

Hemorrhagic fever viruses including Ebola, dengue,
Argentine, and others constitute a group of highly assaultive
diseases that cause severe internal bleeding and, often,
death. Although they have existed for thousands of years in
animals, and in rare cases in humans, only in the past several decades have these viruses been identified by medical
scientists, who developed the reagents necessary to isolate
and identify them. Partly as a result, the numbers of cases
reported have increased.[78]

Hemorrhagic fevers are not exclusive to developing
countries. The 1993 outbreak of Hanta virus pulmonary
syndrome (named after the Hanta River in Korea, where it
was originally discovered) in Arizona showed that the
United States and other developed countries are also at risk
of changing ecological patterns that can induce outbreaks.
After the initial cases were reported and several Navaho
Indians died, CDC scientists found that the vector was a
rural deermouse, *Peromyscus maniculatus*, which is native to
most of North America, including the American southwest.
Apparently, the mouse harbored a strain of the Hanta virus
that causes severe damage to the pulmonary tract and lungs.
It was not clear, however, why this normally reclusive animal had suddenly begun to appear—and leave its droppings—in people's kitchens and playgrounds.[79]

While the highly trained medical detectives failed to
notice that the environment was changing as well as the
pathogens, Navajo medicine men pieced together the expla-
nation for the outbreak. They observed that, prior to the
outbreak, melted snow cascading down to the valley desert
below, combined with heavy spring rains, reminded their
elders of the years 1918 and 1933, when there had been similarly unpredictable weather. In each of those years, disease
had erupted.[80]

In 1992, piñon trees produced an abundance of pine nuts. Descending on the extraordinary harvest, mice had reproduced 10-fold in one season. The rains had then forced the rodents out of their flooded homes and burroughs to scurry about above ground, looking for food and shelter, and increasing exposure to humans. The Navajos understood that when strange symptoms appear, they are not an anomaly. "When there is disharmony in the world, death follows," said one of the medicine men.[81]

Pressures of increasing populations drive many changes in land use, and consequently, outbreaks of infectious disease. Intense human population pressures in Thailand, Vietnam, and southern China, for instance, have generated a shift from diverse family farms to areas of intense, usually, one- or two-crop, agriculture that act like disease zones, where infections can spread rapidly among plants, animals, and humans.[82]

Endemic in many areas of Asia, Japanese encephalitis is expanding its distribution due to increasing demands on farmers to feed ever-growing human populations. When the rice fields are flooded, mosquitoes that are vectors for Japanese encephalitis breed quickly. The rapidly growing numbers of mosquitoes search out new blood and species to feed on. They can infect and be infected by water birds, pigs, and humans. Thus, with rice cultivation, the mosquito vector is introduced, the wading birds arrive, and the virus transmission cycle begins.[83]

When unimmunized farmers go into these areas to cultivate and harvest the rice, many of them are bitten by infected mosquitoes. Every year, more than 30,000 people contract Japanese encephalitis while working in the rice paddies across Asia. Most cases, however, are asymptomatic, or latent. In most endemic countries an active vaccination campaign is in place.[84]

In some cases, animals that serve as microbial hosts and vectors move to new areas, which leads to an outbreak. Essentially, this is what happened in 1973. A new disease (with symptoms resembling flu and arthritis) was identified in Old Lyme, Connecticut, a wooded community near New York City. Like a set of Russian dolls that stack inside one another to make one large doll, a series of environmental disruptions contributed to changes in animal populations which eventually led to an outbreak of Lyme disease.[85]

Deer and mouse populations increased around Old Lyme early in the 1970s, when their natural predators, such as bears and wolves, were driven out and deer hunting was restricted. *Ixodes* ticks, the vectors for the Lyme disease bacterium (*Borrelia*), live and grow in mouse fur. When a tick bites a person, the bacterium moves from the tick's saliva into the victim's bloodstream. Mice and deer then transmit the tick carrying the microbe. So these animals help determine the prevalence of disease.[86]

Since the early 1970s, Lyme disease has spread throughout the United States—due in part to growing numbers of mice, deer, and ticks. It is especially rampant in New England, Wisconsin, and Minnesota, where people live and spend time in wooded areas close to deer populations. In 1994, more than 13,000 cases were reported in the U.S. Cases of other tick-borne infections and rabies (a viral infection that is carried by wild animals but is not tick-borne) have been on the rise in areas of the United States and Europe, as vector populations increase and people move into previously wooded or wilderness areas.[87]

Often, natural disturbances such as heat waves, floods, storms, or earthquakes create the right conditions for microbial traffic, and then the human response in some way magnifies the effects of such disturbances. For example, some experts believe the outbreak of plague in Surat, India, in September 1994 was connected to the flooding of the Tapti River that summer, and to an earthquake a year earlier. The quake hit in 1993, leaving the landscape devastated and thousands homeless. Emergency aid and medical supplies were flown in for the survivors; the appeal for aid was so successful that there was actually too much food. Excess supplies were stored in warehouses, where rats feasted, and then reproduced quickly. The fleas that infest the rodents' fur carried the plague bacterium (*Yersinia pestis*). During the following summer, India was hit by an intense heat wave, with temperatures reaching 51 degrees Celsius (124 degrees Farenheit). Fleas swarmed to animals that had collapsed from the heat.[88]

Then a monsoon flooded the Tapti River and inundated the poorest districts of Surat with three meters of water. Again, people were forced to leave their homes. The rodents were also driven to seek shelter on drier land. Rats and people crowded together on the same high ground, increasing human exposure to the plague bacterium. Although India was medically prepared to deal with waterborne diseases such as gastroenteritis and cholera, and with vector-borne diseases such as malaria, it had no plans for plague. And many doctors who could diagnose and treat plague (which had not been seen in India in several decades) fled the area.[89]

The highly trained medical detectives failed to notice that the environment was changing as well as the pathogens.

The combination of weather patterns and environmental damage from the earthquake and flood were exacerbated by social factors: squalid living conditions in shantytowns and inadequate health care. Media coverage that focused on the disaster without explaining its causes fanned fear into hysteria. What could have been prevented or controlled at an early stage became a financial as well as a social disaster, as international airline flights to and from India were canceled and trade came temporarily to a halt. As a result of the plague, an estimated $2 billion in airline and hotel revenue was lost. Afterwards, mosquitoes proliferated in the monsoon-prone area, and major upsurges of malaria and dengue fever followed. And still, the message of the outbreak—that a rapid and effective surveillance system and trained medical workers are vital to protecting the health of a community—remains unheeded in India and elsewhere.[90]

One reason that prevention in connection with environmental disturbances is underrated is that reliable data linking land use changes to disease outbreaks are rare. What evidence exists tends to be anecdotal and by no means comprehensive. Therefore, epidemiological studies that quantify the link between environmental disruption and the emergence of infectious diseases are badly needed.

In selected cases, data linking effects of water projects, logging, and road building to changes in disease incidence are available, such as the examples of manmade malaria noted earlier. A survey in four states along the Trans-Amazonian Highway by the Brazilian Ministry of Health in 1976 found that the prevalence of malaria was between two and ten times greater within the area of the project than in areas farther away. By clearing forested areas to make room for the highway, people came into places where mosquitoes—the vectors for malaria—had previously fed on other hosts. Subsequently, the infection spread among workers.[91]

Similarly, over the past several decades, the Honduran landscape has been transformed by deforestation, overgrazing, and intense sugarcane and cotton agriculture. Between 1964 and 1990, Honduras lost 34 percent of its pine and deciduous forests through large-scale logging and the cutting of wood for fuel. Deforestation is continuing at an estimated rate of 80,000 hectares annually. Road construction and housing settlements also have disrupted the environment. These land use practices have altered regional rainfall and temperature patterns and affected soil fertility to such a degree that floods and landslides are now more common. Deprived of habitat, sustenance, and blood meals from natural prey, microbes have shifted to infecting humans. Cases of malaria and other vectorborne infectious diseases are on the rise. Twenty thousand cases of malaria were reported in Honduras in 1987, and 90,000 cases were predicted by the end of 1994.[92]

Global climate change is certain to cause disruptions and alterations in the environment. More floods, storms, and droughts are likely, along with changes in rainfall and precipitation. Although it is difficult to predict the exact effects, biological systems and, consequently, human health, are almost sure to be adversely affected.

According to a consensus of the scientific community, global carbon emissions and other trends demonstrate that climate change will become a serious threat to biological stability in the near future. Changes in climate are just beginning to show their effects on environmental systems. Global energy policies have committed the planet's biological system to a certain course of action without regard to its side effects. This trend is largely irreversible, unless immediate and across-the-board cuts are made in emissions from fossil fuels and ozone-depleting chemicals.

In late 1995, Working Group II of the Intergovernmental Panel on Climate Change (IPCC) issued, as part of its larger volume on global impacts, a draft assessment on human health and climate change. The Summary for Policymakers states that "Human-induced climate change represents an important additional stress, particularly to the many ecological and socioeconomic systems already affected by . . . non-sustainable management practices."[93]

A number of variables affect microbes and their vectors. Rates of sexual reproduction and development, the time between feeding cycles, and habitat are sensitive to temperature, humidity, and rainfall. Changing weather patterns, such as heat and heavy flooding, can produce the right environmental conditions for an outbreak of infectious disease. And as these changes become more common, the geographical distribution of microbes will shift. Disease will likely occur when parasites move into "new," previously unexposed areas. For example, major upsurges of dengue in some nations, such as Colombia in 1995, follow periods of heavy rain. And outbreaks of plague in Surat, India, mosquito-borne Ross River Virus (RRV) in coastal southwest Australia, Hanta virus in the southwestern United States, and red tides (toxic phytoplankton) in coastal areas worldwide have been linked to extreme temperature and climatic events.[94]

Risks resulting from changing climate are especially great just outside of current endemic areas or at higher altitudes within endemic areas, and among people who lack immunity. Michael Loevinsohn of the International Development Research Center in New Delhi measured a 337 percent rise in incidence of malaria in Rwanda between 1984 and 1987. The project detected a 1-degree Celsius increase in average temperature during that time period. Heavy rains occurred in 1987, while non-climate variables remained stable. Higher-altitude, mountainous regions of Rwanda, where malaria had previously been "rare or absent," reported a 500 percent increase, compared with 300 percent in lower-lying areas. These findings suggest a link among weather changes, expanding mosquito ranges, and rising malaria incidence.[95]

Research on the mosquito *Culex tarsalis*, the primary vector for Western equine encephalitis and St. Louis encephalitis, has related timing of mosquito development to temperature. Encephalitis is a vector-borne disease whose symptoms vary in severity from mild, flu-like reactions, including high fevers, to fatal inflammation of the brain. In warm weather, mosquito larvae (and encephalitis viruses) breed and mature faster, so the total number of vectors can increase rapidly. Also, the mosquitoes are smaller, and they require more frequent blood meals. When mosquitoes bite humans and animals more often, transmission of encephalitis increases. However, when temperatures are too high, mosquito larvae do not mature. Warmer weather generally increases the transmission of mosquito-borne infections, but only up to a certain threshold temperature.[96]

The Dutch National Institute of Public Health and Environmental Protection reports that a global mean temperature rise of 3 degrees Celsius in 2100 would double the epidemic potential of mosquito populations in tropical regions and would increase it in temperate regions more than 10 times. This means that ecological conditions conducive to malaria would exist in 60 percent, as opposed to the current 45 percent, of the world's land area.[97]

The Institute's model, which examines interactions among climate, mosquitoes, and humans, projects several million more annual malaria cases by 2100. Worldwide, an additional million people could die annually as a result of "the impact of a human-induced climate change on malaria transmission" in the next 60 years.[98]

Changes in temperature and rainfall would also affect the incidence of schistosomiasis, a snail-borne parasitic disease. Although less sensitive to climate change than malaria, schistosomiasis might well expand enough to increase the world population at risk by 0.1 to 1.3 percent (200,000 to 2.6 million), depending on which climate model is used. Some areas, of course, would see case rates decline, while others would become endemic for the first time.[99]

A global mean temperature rise of 3 degrees Celsius in 2100 would double the epidemic potential of mosquito populations in tropical regions.

The same models and technologies that have helped scientists to understand climate change also may help in the control and management of its effects. As Paul Epstein of Harvard University, contributing author of the IPCC health chapter, points out, "While predicting outbreaks of 'new' diseases is not possible, improved prediction of conditions conducive for the resurgence of established vector-borne diseases and waterborne diseases may be more feasible. Improvements in the prediction of climate variability and global linkages of weather patterns could help to generate health early warning systems." Similar calls for microbial traffic planning and tracking centers have been made by Stephen Morse, WHO officials, and others.[100]

Weather forecasting is already integrated with farming and agricultural planning. By applying it to estimates of health risk and extending the forecasting to monitor longer-term climate trends, scientists could model the effects of climate on the epidemiological environment. Combined with remote sensing to map animal and vector habitats, human settlements, and bodies of water, these models could help public officials and decision makers to anticipate health effects and better target prevention efforts.[101]

In the future, along with keeping ecosystems intact and minimizing habitat alterations, communities should require planners to prepare for all the likely consequences of development and to integrate considerations of human health into major human activities such as canal building and farming. And they would do well to provide ongoing health education for their populations, especially in areas that are particularly vulnerable to environmental disruption.

Waterborne Killers

Nearly half of the population in developing countries suffer from health problems associated with water. Eighty percent of all disease in developing countries is spread by unsafe water. In these relatively poor regions, waterborne pathogens and pollution kill between 10 and 25 million people every year—a toll that amounts to one-third of all developing-country deaths.[102]

The waterborne diseases that do most of the killing—diseases such as malaria, cholera, and typhoid—are today primarily tropical: three-quarters of the victims they claim live in the tropics. But to some degree, every population on earth is threatened by waterborne disease. Globally, about 250 million new cases of waterborne infection are reported every year.[103]

This tragedy has its roots in two very basic and common social problems: lack of clean drinking water, and lack of sanitation. (See Figures 3 and 4.) Of course, these problems are closely related: in communities without adequate sanitation, pathogen-laden human and animal wastes, food, and garbage pile up near homes or drain into waterways to infect drinking supplies. A whole range of diarrheal diseases is transmitted through this fecal-oral route: hepatitis A, typhoid fever, cholera, salmonella—even roundworms. In 1993, more than 1.8 billion cases of diarrhea were reported worldwide, predominantly in Sub-Saharan Africa. This is down from nearly 3 billion diarrheal episodes in 1985, thanks to the use of inexpensive rehydration salts.[104]

While we may take it for granted that dirty water is not good for us, this awareness was not always present. During a cholera outbreak in London in 1854, for example, most people blamed their suffering on the rotting garbage in the streets or invisible germs in the air. Then a local doctor named John Snow succeeded in tracing the infection to contaminated drinking water.[105]

That conceptual breakthrough opened the way for one of the most significant public health improvements the world had ever seen—the installation of comprehensive urban sewage systems in western Europe and the United States. By the late nineteenth century, improvements in water supply and sewage systems were having a dramatic effect on urban public health in these areas. In French cities, for example, such improvements helped increase life expectancy from about 32 years in 1850 to about 45 years by 1900.[106]

And yet, more than a century after Snow's discovery, we have not managed to find a way to break the grip of cholera and other waterborne diseases on much of the developing world. Globally, having enough clean water to drink and bathe in is a life or death issue for one out of every five people.[107]

To become infected, all a person may need is a drink, a swim, or a meal of contaminated fish. For example, an outbreak of cholera that began in Peru in 1991—its first appearance in Latin America after more than 60 years—gradually contaminated the water supplies of every country in that continent except for Paraguay and Uruguay, infecting more than 500,000 people before it subsided two years later. The region lost more than $750 million from seafood kept from export because of cholera. The Pan American Health

FIGURE 3

Share of Population with Safe Drinking Water, by Region, 1990

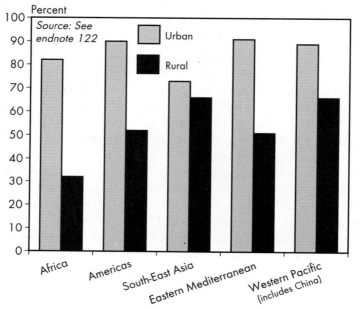

Organization estimated that it will take more than a decade and $200 billion to control the damage caused by this latest cholera outbreak.[108]

Prior to the cholera epidemic, most countries in Latin America and the Caribbean had focused on the quantity of water available, rather than its quality. Fewer than 25 percent of community water systems in Latin America were "reliably and continuously disinfected." The disease got around the ordinary preventive measures, such as boiling drinking water, because many people were consuming the bacterium (*Vibrio cholerae*) by eating *ceviche*, raw fish with lemon juice. As a result of the epidemic, many countries focused more on water quality issues and initiated public education campaigns. The success was incredible: by using oral rehydration therapy (ORT), Peruvian doctors and nurses kept the mortality rate to one percent.[109]

FIGURE 4

Share of Population with Adequate Sanitation, by Region, 1990

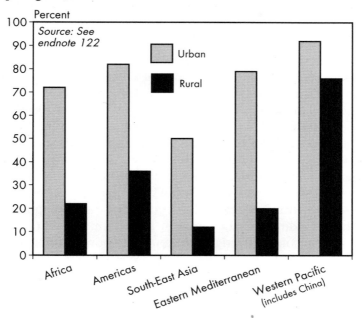

At the same time that cholera reappeared in Latin America, a new strain, *V. cholerae* 0139, emerged in India and Bangladesh. First detected in Madras in late 1992, this strain spread to other South Asian countries six months later; Bangladesh was hit the worst. At the peak of the epidemic in Dhaka, 600 people became sick every day. By the time the epidemic finished its rampage through Calcutta's water supplies, more than 15,000 people were infected and 230 had died. The epidemic eventually struck more than a million people across South Asia and killed at least 10,000.[110]

While the South Asian epidemic has since burned out, traces of cholera 0139 still exist in the environment and it is likely that still newer strains of cholera will crop up in response to environmental pressures. The cholera bacterium can essentially hibernate with algae hosts for extended periods of time and then emerge seasonally, when temperature, sunlight, nutrient levels, and acidity are adequate for its survival.[111]

Human development activities, especially dams and irrigation projects, can exacerbate the spread of waterborne infectious diseases. Richard Toll, a Senegalese town 370 kilometers northeast of Dakar, literally means Richard's "Field" in the local Wallof language, conjuring up images of lush when green land. But it was not until 1985, when the Daima Dam was built along the Senegal River by the Mauritanian, Senegalese, and Malian governments, that the town lived up to its name. Harnessing the river's water made it possible to transform 10,000 hectares of desert soil into fields of sugarcane, potatoes, mint, and even rice. The irrigated area eventually grew to 40,000 hectares and a few members of the local Wallof tribe became millionaires.[112]

Along with jobs came infectious disease, as happened with the Indira Gandhi Canal in Rajasthan. Sanitation in the area is poor and irrigation canals are now infected with strains of diarrheal bacteria. People have no choice but to drink the water, wash their laundry in it, and bathe in it. The government has shown no willingness to spend the money necessary to provide people with a clean water supply.[113]

Another consequence of the dam project was to halt the daily influx of saltwater from the Atlantic Ocean that flowed up the Senegal River almost 200 kilometers inland. Seasonal and daily fluctuations of the water level had kept snails to a minimum, but after the dam was built, this natural check ceased. The dam created prefect conditions for an epidemic of snail-borne schistosomiasis.

With a constant and relatively calm supply of fresh water, snails quickly populated the canals and river. The first case of intestinal schistosomiasis was detected in 1988; two years later, about 60 percent of the population exhibited symptoms—bloody urine and stools, vomiting, diarrhea, fever, cough, and internal organ swelling. In a survey of Ndombo, a village that had prospered from mint crops made possible by the dam, 91 percent of the people were infected.[114]

The situation in Richard Toll may get worse before it improves: a Belgian research group has identified another snail that carries yet another form of schistosomiasis in nearby canals. It can cause cirrhosis of the liver and, in rare cases, bladder cancer in people; it also infects and kills livestock.[115]

Epidemics of schistosomiasis are nothing new. Egyptian mummies that date back to 1200 B.C. still have eggs of its pathogen, the blood fluke *Schistosoma*. Also known as bilharzia-sis, this disabling disease was common in areas of China around 200 B.C., during the Han Dynasty, a time of expanding rice cultivation along the Yellow River.[116]

Schistosomiasis continues to be a major killer in the twentieth century.

Globally, having enough clean water to drink and bathe in is a life or death issue for one out of every five people.

It is the second leading tropical disease after malaria. Annually, between 150 and 200 million people are at risk of contracting schistosomiasis, and 200,000 people die from it. The disease is endemic to certain parts of Africa, Asia, and South America, where it infects farmers and fishers who spend a lot of time wading through the shallow waters favored by the snails. The cycle of transmission continues when people defecate the larvae, which then travel through water supplies and infect other snails or people.[117]

Other diseases work variations on the same theme. Diseases (such as malaria, dengue, yellow fever, Japanese encephalitis) rely on water for part of their life cycles. Onchocerciasis, or river blindness, for instance, afflicts some 18 million people predominantly in West Africa, especially in Cameroon and Nigeria, as well as scattered regions in Latin America and the Eastern Mediterranean. This organ-ism is carried by a blackfly that breeds along the regions' rapid-moving streams and causes severe skin lesions, der-matitis, and eye lesions; about 10 percent of the cases result in blindness. In Sub-Saharan Africa, people have left the areas traversed by such streams for fear of this fly.[118]

The lack of clean water has generated the familiar image of African and Asian women balancing jugs on their heads—a reminder that the burden of collecting water falls primarily on women. In Nigeria's Imo state, for example, the average household invests six hours a day collecting water during the dry season. The long walk out, the queue at the source, and the hard trek home cut deeply into time that could be spent in school or at other productive work.[119]

Often, government intervention fails to reach those who need it most. Government-owned water utilities may provide services only to landowners or homeowners, so the large squatter populations typical of many cities may fall outside the scope of the service. A family in the top fifth income group in Peru, the Dominican Republic, or Ghana is, respectively, three, six, or twelve times more likely to have a house water connection than a family in the bottom fifth. Rural areas are especially underserved.[120] (See Figure 3.)

But access to safe drinking water is only half the problem. Without safe ways to store clean water, and safe ways to dispose of used water, any progress made up to the tap can be quickly undone. Sometimes new community supplies actually contribute to the spread of disease. In crowded urban areas, for example, seepage around hand pumps and storage facilities can create breeding sites for the mosquitoes that carry dengue, yellow fever, and malaria.[121]

Of course, sewage presents an even graver disease potential. In 1990, an estimated 1.7 billion people worldwide threw their sewage out untreated. The situation in rural areas of developing countries is particularly troubling. In the African countryside, only one out of five people is served by an appropriate means of sanitation, and in rural Southeast Asia, only a meager 12 percent of the population have minimal sanitation facilities. (See Figures 4.) Even the simplest arrangements, such as outdoor latrines or sewage pits, can make an enormous difference. In households lacking such facilities, children have a 60 percent higher chance of dying from diarrhea. To help reverse this situation, households can use solar cookers and other energy-efficient devices to clean water of most pathogens.[122]

In more densely populated areas, of course, waste management becomes a more complex affair. Many of the urban sewage systems in the developing, and former East Bloc, countries, for instance, are simply not up to the demands placed upon them. Crumbling sanitation systems have turned the region's rivers into sewers. Three-fourths of Poland's rivers are so contaminated by chemicals, sewage, and agricultural runoff that their water is unfit even for industrial use. Nearly half of the water and sewage treatment systems in Moscow are ineffective or malfunctioning.[123]

After years of infrastructure decay and a breakdown in government monitoring of water standards, 75 percent of the Russian Republic's lake and river water is unsafe to drink because of bacterial contamination. In a single year, January 1992 to January 1993, Russia's incidence of bacterial dysentery jumped 128 percent. (Bacterial dysentery is a group of diseases that cause intestinal pain and bloody diarrhea; cholera is among the most severe of these.) During the same time, Russia saw its typhoid infections grow by 300 percent. In May 1994, cholera appeared in Moscow, evidently travelling north from the Black Sea coast, where it had been detected in plankton several months earlier.[124]

In more developed countries, better sewage treatment and other pollution-control technologies keep the contamination of inland surface waters fairly low by comparison. These measures, combined with chlorination of drinking water—which is standard practice in Europe, North America, and Japan—have also greatly reduced the possibility of waterborne infection. But even in the richest countries, serious problems remain.

In the United States, for example, deaths from waterborne infectious diseases have declined dramatically since monitoring began in the early twentieth century. Cases of typhoid and cholera are nearly unheard of in the U.S. today.

However, in the past 30 to 40 years, the number of cases of contagious waterborne disease have increased, especially cryptosporidiosis and various viral infections. Every year more than 700,000 Americans contract cryptosporidiosis, an infection by a waterborne protozoan that causes prolonged diarrhea, abdominal pain, weight loss, and fever. The pathogen, *Cryptosporidium*, is extremely difficult to exclude from water supplies because a very low number can cause infection and it is often resistant to disinfectants at levels acceptable in drinking water.[125]

A survey in 1992 showed that nearly 40 percent of treated drinking water supplies in the United States contained either *Cryptosporidium* or *Giardia*, a pathogen that infects the small intestine. The infection, giardiasis, causes a wide range of symptoms including nausea, diarrhea, weight loss and lethargy. Cryptosporidium has also been reported in England and The Netherlands. One study noted that nearly one-third of all cases of diarrhea in North America can be associated with consuming inadequately treated drinking water.[126]

The economic costs of these cases are significant. Analysis by the U.S. Environmental Protection Agency estimates that waterborne infectious diseases annually cost the nation about $1.6 billion (in 1991 dollars) for an estimated 560,000 moderate-to-severe cases, and an additional $20.3 billion for an estimated 7.1 million mild-to-moderate cases.[127]

It should come as no surprise that keeping water supplies clean requires continuous effort. Protecting water quality is our first line of defense for human and ecological health. But technology alone cannot solve the problems associated with water quality—it also takes environmental protection. On this front, much can be learned from water protection measures in Brazil's Guarapiranga water basin. These measures recognize the importance of protecting the river system—the floodplains, creeks, wild life, fisheries, and watershed—and its natural recuperative powers. In the near future, environmental education projects will be set up to promote sustainable fishing and farming.[128]

Successful solutions are often based on simple techniques—such as public education and local stewardship—not expensive technology. During the 1980s, for example, WHO launched a series of locally based education campaigns in Africa to prevent Guinea worm disease. Also known as dracunculiasis, this infection is caused by a protozoan that is transmitted by a water flea, *Cyclops*. When people drink infected water, the protozoan enters the bloodstream and, over the course of a year, matures into a worm up to a meter long. As the worm grows inside the body, it causes the disease that blisters the skin. Because the blisters feel as if they're burning, victims often submerge their legs and arms in water to cool them off. Eventually, the worm emerges through the victim's skin and releases new larvae into the water, thus continuing the deadly cycle of infection.[129]

Technology alone cannot solve the problems associated with water quality—it also takes environmental protection.

Fortunately, it is relatively easy to prevent Guinea worm disease. Health education programs focus on teaching people how to filter drinking water to remove the larvae and then to boil or chlorinate the water as a further precaution. By learning how to ward off infection in the first place, people have lowered the incidence of Guinea worm dramatically in recent years as a result of WHO's eradication campaign: from 3.5 million cases in 1986 to less than 100,000 in 1995. WHO officials predict that this debilitating disease could be eradicated from the globe within the next decade.[130]

There are equally simple techniques for handling other types of infections as well. For example, cholera and dysentery deaths can be reduced by as much as 80 percent with oral rehydration therapy—an inexpensive mixture of water, sugar, and salt that is given to diarrhea patients as soon as they can drink. In Sub-Saharan Africa, UNICEF has been working with families directly, supplying them with the ORT mixture and showing them how to use it. Of course, not all diseases can be treated this easily, but the potential of this technique is enormous. In 1993 alone, ORT saved more than 1 million children's lives throughout the developing world. (Yet, 2.5 million children still died from untreated diarrheal diseases.) If implemented widely, such relatively simple programs could radically improve the lives of millions of people.[131]

Wonder Drugs No More

The protozoa responsible for malaria, *Plasmodium*, have a long history of stopping human armies in their tracks. Malaria, one of the most deadly infections known to humankind, prevented European explorers from venturing far inland in Africa. British soldiers in India in the 1850s had firsthand knowledge of the disease; and more than 1.2 million Union soldiers succumbed to it during the United States Civil War when they marched south. Malaria and yellow fever also kept the French from building the first Panama Canal.[132]

By 1960, with the development of chloroquine and the employment of insecticides such as DDT, WHO felt able to predict malaria's elimination. Nevertheless, this disease has made a recent comeback with the evolution of drug-resistant strains of *Plasmodium*. At an American penny a dose, chloroquine was prescribed like aspirin in some African countries to treat malaria symptoms. By the late 1960s, chloroquine-resistant *Plasmodium falciparum* had evolved in South America and Southeast Asia. By the late 1970s, these strains had spread through Asia, India, the Middle East, and East Africa, and over the next 10 years they swept west across Sub-Saharan Africa.[133]

Today, almost all disease-causing bacteria are on the pathway to complete drug resistance. More than a half century after the discovery of antibiotics, humanity is at risk of losing these valuable weapons and reverting to the pre-antibiotic era.

Alexander Fleming's discovery of the antibacterial properties of *Penicillium* mold in 1929 led to enormous progress in controlling the threat and incidence of infectious diseases in the 1940s and 1950s. With a growing arsenal of therapeutic drugs—including penicillin, tetracycline, and ampicillin—WHO, national governments, and medical authorities initiated campaigns to wipe infectious diseases from the face of the earth. By the 1970s, however, the optimism and expectations of earlier years were tempered by the realization that antibiotics are tools that can only control microbes when used effectively—and sparingly. Still, improper use of these drugs has continued to grow.[134]

The misuse of antibiotics seems surprising in view of the fact that Fleming urged caution early on in his work. In the lab, he derived mutant bacteria by using progressively higher amounts of penicillin and showed that the drug could not penetrate the mutant bacteria cell walls. He feared that penicillin would be misused if it became available in oral form. In 1945, he said:

> *"The greatest possibility of evil in self-medication is the use in too small doses so that instead of clearing up infection, the microbes are educated to resist penicillin and a host of penicillin-fast organisms is bred out which can be passed to other individuals and from them to others until they reach someone who gets a septicemia or a pneumonia which penicillin cannot save."*[135]

From a public health perspective, incomplete or interrupted treatment of infection poses a greater threat than non-treatment because it encourages strains of drug-resistant bacteria. When an antibiotic is used incorrectly, some of the organisms survive the initial dose. They become immune or resistant to the drug, and then reproduce. Gradually they become the dominant strain of the microbe, and the antibiotics lose their effectiveness. Resistant strains develop particularly fast when doctors overuse antibiotics and try to eliminate the bacteria rather than control them. If 99.9 percent are killed, the survivors are likely to be a superstrain.[136]

"Antibiotics are societal drugs," observes Stuart Levy, a specialist in drug resistance. Antibiotic-resistant bacteria are often shed and excreted into the environment at large, where they can become a widespread problem. Once drug-resistant mutants evolve, they never disappear.[137]

By 1955, most countries recognized the problem of overuse and restricted the use of penicillin by requiring prescriptions. But this was not enough to stop massive overuse of antibiotics. In 1992, U.S. doctors prescribed these drugs 28 percent more than they did in 1980. It is not simply the sheer number of antibiotics, but how they are used and applied that creates problems. Of the 150 million antibiotic prescriptions written every year by American doctors, almost half are misprescribed or misused. Some antibiotics are prescribed for viral infections, upon which they have no effect. Other times symptoms are simply misdiagnosed or doctors give in to patients' requests for pills, or recommended treatment is not followed properly. Worldwide, an estimated $9 billion is wasted every year because of irrational use of these drugs.[138]

A high portion of antibiotics—about half—are used for livestock, aquaculture, and other biological industries. They are administered with growth hormones to prevent illness in breeding sites, such as fish and animal farms throughout the world.[139]

Monocultural farming is a major source of the drug resistance problem. When farms harvest just one crop or raise a large number of one kind of animal, the conditions are ripe for disease outbreak. A commercial chicken farm may house 100,000 chickens for instance; an aquaculture facility may breed thousands of salmon or tilapia. When an infectious disease occurs in a monoculture like these, it can sweep through a farm, killing many of the animals. It also may spread to other populations, just as influenza strains can cross from poultry and pigs to humans.[140]

First reported in New Guinea in 1967, antibiotic-resistant *Streptococcus pneumoniae*, which causes a range of infections, including pneumonia and the often fatal blood infection septicemia, is a leading cause of sickness and even death among young children and the elderly worldwide. Drug-resistant pneumococcal infections became common in South Africa in the 1970s, Europe in the 1980s, and the United States in the 1990s. Throughout Europe in 1979, only 6 percent of pneumococcus strains were penicillin resistant; by 1989, this number had grown to 44 percent. A case study in Atlanta, Georgia, reported that 41 percent of pneumococcal infections in children under age six were resistant to penicillin by 1994.[141]

In the United States, more than 90 percent of staphylococcus strains now resist treatment by penicillin. Some pneumococcal infections, as well as the closely related staphylococcal and streptococcal infections—which cause high fever, sore throat, earaches, and pneumonia—are resistant to every antibiotic except one: vancomycin. It is just a matter of time before this drug also becomes ineffective. Rare enterococcal infections—which infect surgical wounds, as well as the urinary tract, heart, and bloodstream—are already resistant to vancomycin. Enterococci will eventually transfer the vancomycin-resistant material to other, more common infections. Resistance to vancomycin increased 40 times between 1989 and 1993, from 0.3 percent to more than 13 percent of enterococcal infections in intensive-care units of hospitals, according to a surveillance program run by CDC. (See Figure 5.)[142]

At this time, drug-resistant infections are not necessarily more dangerous to the patient, but they are more difficult, and sometimes more expensive, to treat. The annual cost of treating infections that are resistant to more than one drug is $100 to $200 million in the United States. Annually, Americans pay more than $4 billion in drug-resistance-related medical costs for bacterial infections, according to the

Centers for Disease Control and Prevention. Doctors increasingly have to prescribe longer hospital stays, alternative treatments, and more toxic and expensive drugs as strains of disease resistant to single and multiple medicines become more common.[143]

Fortunately, it is possible to reverse this trend. In Iceland, the first case of penicillin-resistant S. pneumoniae was detected in 1988 at a hospital in Reykjavik; three years later, 20 percent of the country's cases were resistant to penicillin. But with government-monitored drug use, nationwide screening of pneumococcal infections, and massive publicity and education drives, the situation was reversed. Doctors were advised to observe patients closely and monitor symptoms as they progressed, rather than resorting to drug treatment, especially in the event of an uncertain diagnosis or a mild infection. As a result of these efforts, infections had declined from 20 percent to 17 percent of cases by 1994. Among children at daycare centers, the decline was even greater. Although the results may not be statistically significant as yet, Iceland's experience demonstrates that modified use of drug use reverses the increase in drug resistance.[144]

Health clinics and doctors everywhere can safeguard the antibiotics that still work by using them sparingly and making sure that patients use them as prescribed. CDC recommends that hospitals regularly test for vancomycin-resistant enterococci and isolate patients who have this infection.[145]

Another strategy is to avoid using antibiotics in the first place and to emphasize prevention of infectious disease rather than treatment. Vaccinations can help control illness by reducing the need for so many drugs. Boosting individual immunity improves not only individual health, but also the health of the population at large. Increasing the number of immune individuals reduces the chances of an infection spreading unchecked through the population.

One way to become immune to illness is to survive an infection. After contracting a particular disease, immunity specific to it follows. Immunizations stimulate the immune

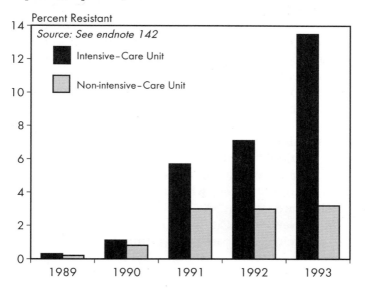

FIGURE 5

Incidence of Vancomycin-Resistant Enterococci in U.S. Hospitals, by Year, 1989–1993

system to produce the antibody, just as it would in response to the real infection. Immunization is not a complete protection against infection or death, however; there is still a small chance that the individual will get sick.[146]

A campaign by UNICEF during the 1970s and 1980s significantly reduced many infectious diseases by providing widespread immunization. By 1990, a full 80 percent of the world's children had received immunizations for lethal diseases, including diphtheria, pertussis, tetanus, typhoid, and polio, up from 25 percent in 1980. The measles vaccine alone reduced childhood deaths from 2.5 million in 1980 to less than 900,000 only 10 years later. Vaccines administered in 1992 saved 3 million children's lives worldwide. Another 1.7 million deaths could have been prevented with even wider coverage.[147]

Because no magic bullet exists to control infectious disease, constant vigilance is necessary. In 1993, just 26 years after Dr. Stewart made his proclamation of victory, another former U.S. Surgeon General, C. Everett Koop, wrote, "ironically, in conquering these (polio and measles) and other potentially deadly diseases, we have inadvertently created a misplaced sense of complacency." Clearly, we need to reopen the book on infectious disease and reexamine our thinking.[148]

Even after years of experience with mass immunizations, the American national average immunization rate is only 58 percent, far below the rates in many developing countries, including Mexico, Thailand, India, and Uganda. An estimated 3 million American children are not immunized against traditional childhood infections. The children who suffer from these easily prevented diseases are many of the nation's poorest children, who "fall through the cracks" of the health care system. A 1994 study found that only 24 percent of New York City children on Medicaid received standard vaccines compared to a pitiful citywide average of 49 percent.[149]

In the United States, county and city health officials are now teaming up with McDonald's fast-food restaurant to circulate back-to-school immunization reminders. In Harlem, volunteers with the Hope for Kids program—a national effort to immunize inner-city children—welcome winter storms because snow days make it possible to find children and their parents or guardians at home.[150]

While drug resistance is a growing problem, hope may be on the horizon. As in Hungary and Iceland, steps are being taken to slow the proliferation of drug-resistant microbes. And research and development for new vaccines and antibiotics are underway. SPf66, the first vaccine developed against malaria, reduced its incidence by one-third among children, in a test run in Tanzania. Other tests have had similar results, but the vaccine awaits approval by international health officials. Meanwhile, millions of people suffer from all forms of the disease, and the dying continues.[151]

Writing the Prescription

Rarely are the costs of environmental deterioration as clear, the stakes for human well-being as high, or the risks for biological stability as great as in the nexus between microbes and hosts. Here an uneasy balance—between the unseen microscopic environment and the world of plants, animals, and humans—represents a constantly evolving relationship based on mutual coexistence. Today, the growing incidence of infectious disease in large areas of the world indicates that this relationship is in trouble, the result of many collisions between increasing human activity and the planet's physical and biological systems.

As human populations expand and stream toward cities, as species diversity declines at unprecedented rates, as the resilience of land and water systems is further stressed, and global climate patterns shift, the natural world is being profoundly altered. As a result, people—along with plants and animals—are becoming more vulnerable to infectious diseases, including several that seemed to have been conquered long ago.

Some may wonder if microbes are, in effect, nature's ultimate check: pruning populations that expand beyond the ability of the earth to support them. But the evidence suggests otherwise. Eighty-eight million people are being added to the planet each year—more than five times as many people as are killed by infectious diseases. The stabilizing effects of high mortality rates are greatly outweighed by the cumulative negative impacts on society—reduced life expectancy, increased illness, higher health costs, lost productivity—that result when contagious diseases tear through families, communities, and ecosystems.

Therefore, as the global community struggles to write an effective prescription to head off the looming epidemic of epidemics, it is clear that we will need to attack the problem on two levels, by stepping up efforts to address the underlying forces that are driving the recent upward surge in disease, and by addressing the serious inadequacy of health care programs, particularly in developing countries.

Because infectious diseases are a basic barometer of the overall sustainability of human activity, we will have to address the key elements of sustainable economic development in order to ultimately control them. Although these solutions are well beyond the scope of this paper, their basic elements are clear: stabilizing world population, reversing the tide of deforestation, sustainably managing and cleaning up the world's precious supplies of fresh water, and drastically reducing the 25 billion tons of carbon dioxide that are now being added to the atmosphere each year and disrupting the climate.[152]

While it is crucial that the underlying causes of infectious disease be addressed, immediate and specific preventive measures, the nuts-and-bolts of public health, can do much to reduce the numbers of people suffering and dying. In the short term, governments, the medical community, and individuals can improve vaccination campaigns; expand public health education programs; limit the use of antibiotics and other drugs; and provide basic health services and care. One of the keys to confronting pathogenic microbes is to use the tools we already have in hand more effectively. Of equal importance is to expand access to clean water and health services, and to improve distribution of medicines, vaccines, and educational materials.

The best counter-measure to infection is to build up people's immunity and stop infection before it gets started. Reinvigorating the global push begun in the 1980s by UNICEF and WHO to vaccinate every child, and supporting wide distribution of ORT and other basic public health treatments could go a long way toward controlling the spread of infectious disease. Preventive strategies such as mass vaccination cost little compared with the lives and money they save.

The reasons for not completing immunization routines include language barriers, limited clinic hours, poverty, strife, and ignorance. To circumvent these problems and boost immunity among children, many countries now organize National Immunization Days (NIDs) twice a year. The NID concept has been applied to wartorn areas such as Colombia, El Salvador, Lebanon, and, in 1995, the Sudan. In El Salvador, UNICEF officials negotiated with President Duarte and guerrilla leaders to hold regularly scheduled "days of tranquility" each year. As a result of these temporary cease-fires, Salvadoran children's immunization rates soared from 3 percent in 1984 to 80 percent in 1990, even as civil war raged.[153]

Because so many infections are easily treated, improving medical care, particularly in developing countries, would help to reduce the numbers of infections that develop into severe illness. In addition to promoting prevention and health care, doctors, medical workers, and health officials would do well to test regularly for drug-resistant strains of microbes. To safeguard the antibiotics that still work, it is essential to use them sparingly and under monitored conditions, especially in agricultural settings.

Beyond money for prevention and treatment programs, another prudent use of scarce funding is for biomedical research and ongoing education. Money and political support are needed to revamp research and development of new diagnostic tests, vaccines, medicines, antimicrobial drugs, and more equitable distribution methods, as well as to improve public education,

In the long run, prevention is our most effective weapon against infectious disease.

health clinic outreach programs, and other means to raise public awareness. Even in the 1990s, most doctors in Africa and other developing countries lack routine access to even basic medical equipment. Meanwhile, disease outbreaks can rage for months unattended. Agencies such as WHO and CDC have suffered financial cutbacks that severely limit efforts to respond to and control infectious disease.[154]

Signs of a growing awareness that everyone is potentially at risk include a flurry of recent international efforts aimed at limiting infectious disease. In 1995, the WHO General Assembly passed a resolution urging member states to strengthen surveillance; improve rapid diagnosis, communication, and response; conduct routine testing for drug resistance; and increase the number of skilled staff who can treat infectious diseases.[155]

The worldwide Program for Monitoring Emerging Diseases (ProMED) of people, animals, and plants is an active global computer network that facilitates communication among health workers, scientists, and journalists. Since its inception in August 1994, more than 100 countries and 3,500 individuals have joined ProMED. In May 1995, scientists and health workers regularly logged onto this network to monitor the Ebola outbreak in Kikwit, Zaire, and to receive field reports. In a similar move, members of the European Union established an on-line network in 1994, Salmnet, to track salmonella infections and coordinate response.[156]

Governments can also establish tracking centers to monitor environmental and health trends at global, regional, and local levels. Outposts all over the world reporting back to WHO, or some other coordinating body, will help public health officials understand the life cycles of diseases and respond to outbreaks faster. Better integration of environmental and health monitoring—using satellites, computers, remote sensing, and Geographic Information Systems—can identify the conditions conducive to outbreaks of infectious disease and predict where they are likely to occur. International efforts, such as the IPCC report on global climate change and human health, are setting a precedent for the type of interdisciplinary work that is needed to address infectious diseases.[157]

In the long run, prevention is our most effective weapon against infectious disease: public health measures that improve the health of individuals and populations, as well as sustainable economic and environmental policies that control the emergence and spread of infectious diseases and maintain the natural checks and balances will go a long way toward promoting a healthier world. The price of failing to understand these links is clear: rising health care costs and a world in which, even now, more than half the people live in fear of plagues that are as certain as evolution itself.

Notes

1. Stewart quote from James LeFanu, "Return of the Man-killing Microbes," *Financial Times*, October 28-29, 1995.

2. The Harvard Working Group on New and Resurgent Diseases, "New and Resurgent Diseases: The Failure of Attempted Eradication," *The Ecologist*, January/February 1995; Paul R. Epstein, "Examples of Emerging and Resurgent Infectious Diseases in the 1990s," *Course Reader: Climate Change, Ecology and Public Health*, Harvard University School of Public Health, September 1995; Working Group on Emerging and Re-emerging Infectious Diseases, Committee on International Science, Engineering, and Technology (CISET), *Global Microbial Threats in the 1990s* (Washington, D.C.: National Science and Technology Council, 1995).

3. Director-General, *The World Health Report 1995: Bridging the Gaps* (Geneva: World Health Organization (WHO), 1995); "anything but new" from Stephen S. Morse, "Controlling Infectious Diseases," *Technology Review*, October 1995; Hippocrates from William H. McNeill, *Plagues and People* (Garden City, N.Y.: Anchor Press/Doubleday, 1976).

4. Drug resistance from Director-General, op. cit. note 3; Stuart B. Levy, *The Antibiotic Paradox: How Miracle Drugs Are Destroying the Miracle* (New York: Plenum Press, 1992); CISET, op. cit. note 2.

5. Sir MacFarlane Burnet and David O. White, *Natural History of Infectious Disease*, 4th ed. (Cambridge: Cambridge University Press, 1972); John Maynard Smith, "Bacteria Break the Antibiotic Bank," *Natural History*, June 1994.

6. Beverly E. Griffin, "Live and Let Live," *Nature*, March 3, 1994; Smith, op. cit. note 5.

7. Figure of 1,000 copies from Stephen S. Morse, The Rockefeller University, New York City, private communication, October 17, 1995; human cells from Robin Marantz Henig, *A Dancing Matrix: Voyages Along the Viral Frontier* (New York: Alfred A. Knopf, 1993); Paul R. Epstein, "Commentary: Pestilence and Poverty—Historical Transitions and the Great Pandemics," *American Journal of Preventive Medicine*, Vol. 8, No. 4, 1992.

8. Paul R. Epstein, "Biodiversity: The Diversity of Life," *Journal of the American Medical Association*, April 21, 1993; 13,000 cases from Daniel B. Fishbein and David T. Dennis, "Tick-borne Diseases: A Growing Risk," *The New England Journal of Medicine*, August 17, 1995.

9. Director-General, op. cit. note 3.

10. Joel E. Cohen, "Population Growth and Earth's Human Carrying Capacity," *Science*, July 21, 1995; population data from Aaron Sachs, "Population Growth Steady," in Lester R. Brown, Nicholas Lenssen, and Hal Kane, *Vital Signs 1995* (New York: W.W. Norton & Company, 1995); Elena Wilken, "Urbanization Spreading," in Brown et al., op. cit. this note; Anjali Acharya, "Tropical Forests Vanishing," in Brown et al., op. cit. this note; Extinction rates from Stuart L. Pimm et al., "The Future of Biodiversity," *Science*, July 25, 1995.

11. David Malin Roodman, "Carbon Emissions Resume Rise," in Brown et al., op. cit. note 10.

12. Levy, op. cit. note 4; National Center for Infectious Diseases (NCID), *Addressing Emerging Infectious Disease Threats: A Prevention Strategy for the United States* (Atlanta, Ga.: Centers for Disease Control and Prevention (CDC), 1994).

13. Director-General, op. cit. note 3.

14. CISET, op. cit. note 2; World Bank, *World Development Report 1993: Investing in Health* (New York: Oxford University Press, 1993); Helen Saxenian, "Optimizing Health Care in Developing Countries," *Issues in Science and Technology*, Winter 1994-95; Peter Cowley and Dean T. Jamison, "The Cost-Effectiveness of Immunization," *World Health*, March/April 1993; John Maurice, "Polio Eradication: the Finishing Line in Sight," *Children's Vaccine Initiative (CVI) Forum*, Geneva, June 1995.

15. Rachel Nowak, "Hungary Sees an Improvement in Penicillin Resistance," *Science*, April 15, 1994.

16. CISET, op. cit. note 2; Paul R. Epstein, David J. Rogers, and Rudi Slooff, "Satellite Imaging and Vector-borne Disease," *The Lancet*, May 29, 1993.

17. Population data reflect medium variance of 4.1 billion from United Nations, *World Population Prospects: The 1994 Revision* (New York: 1995); Henrylito D. Tacio, "Poverty is World's Deadliest Disease," *Depthnews*, November 1995; Director-General, op. cit. note 3.

18. Director-General, op. cit. note 3; antibiotic-resistant strains from Stuart B. Levy, Director, Center for Adaptation Genetics and Drug Resistance, Tufts University School of Medicine, Medford, Mass., private communication, June 8, 1995.

19. Director-General, op. cit. note 3; malaria data from WHO, "World Malaria Situation in 1992, Part I: Middle South Asia, Eastern Asia and Oceania," *Weekly Epidemiological Record*, October 21, 1994; Elizabeth J. Taylor, *Dorland's Illustrated Medical Dictionary*, 27th ed. (Philadelphia: W.B. Saunders Company, 1988); "Catalog of Emerging Infectious Disease Agents," Appendix A in Joshua Lederberg, Robert E. Shope, and Stanley C.

Oaks, Jr., eds., *Emerging Infections: Microbial Threats to Health in the United States* (Washington, D.C.: National Academy Press, 1992); Wayne Biddle, *A Field Guide to Germs* (New York: Henry Holt and Co., 1995); *Tropical Disease Research: Progress 1991-92*, Eleventh Program Report of the UNDP/World Bank/WHO Special Program for Research and Training in Tropical Diseases (TDR) (Geneva: WHO, 1993); cholera from Council for Agricultural Science and Technology (CAST), *Foodborne Pathogens: Risks and Consequences*, CAST Task Force Report, No. 122, September 1994.

20. Robert W. Pinner et al., "Trends in Infectious Diseases Mortality in the United States," *The Journal of the American Medical Association*, January 17, 1996.

21. Director-General, op. cit. note 3; Susan Okie, "500 Million Infected With Tropical Ills," *Washington Post*, March 28, 1990; more than 100 infectious diseases from Andrew A. Arata, Vector Biology and Control Project (now the Environmental Health Project), U.S. Agency for International Development, "Impact of Environmental Changes on Endemic Vector-borne Diseases" (paper presented at "Achieving Health for All: Economic and Social Policy," Seattle, Wash., September 10-13, 1989); CAST, op. cit. note 19; Duane J. Gubler, "Vector-Borne Diseases," in Ruth A. Eblen and William R. Eblen, eds., *The Encyclopedia of the Environment* (Boston, Mass.: Houghton Mifflin Company, 1994).

22. Robin A. Weiss, "Darwin and Disease," *Nature*, November 17, 1994; Burnet and White, op. cit. note 5; Louis H. Miller, Michael F. Good, Geneviève Milon, "Malaria Pathogenesis," *Science*, June 24, 1994; Frank H. Collins and Nora J. Besansky, "Vector Biology and the Control of Malaria in Africa," *Science*, June 24, 1994.

23. Smallpox from Laurie Garrett, *The Coming Plague: Newly Emerging Diseases in a World Out of Balance* (New York: Farrar, Straus, and Giroux, 1994); measles from Stanley O. Foster, Deborah A. McFarland, and A. Meredith John, "Measles," in Dean T. Jamison et al., eds., *Disease Control Priorities in Developing Countries* (Washington, D.C.: World Bank, 1993); "Number of Cases of Measles Reported Globally, 1974-1989," *World Health Statistics Quarterly*, Vol. 45, 1992; Reuters, "In Finland, Exit Mumps and Measles," *New York Times*, November 25, 1994.

24. Polio from Dean T. Jamison et al., "Poliomyelitis," in Jamison et al., op. cit. note 23; "Towards a World Without Polio," *World Health*, Special Issue: January/February 1995; Frances Williams, "End to Polio by 2000," *Financial Times*, April 7, 1995.

25. Ruth L. Berkelman, Ralph T. Bryan, Michael T. Osterholm, James W. LeDuc, and James M. Hughes, "Infectious Disease Surveillance: A Crumbling Foundation," *Science*, April 15, 1994; NCID, op. cit. note 12.

26. Director-General, op. cit. note 3.

27. Nigeria from J.M. Meegan, "Yellow Fever Vaccine," *WHO/EPI/General*, Vol. 91, No. 6, 1991, and from T.P. Monath, "Yellow Fever: Victor, Victoria? Conqueror, Conquest? Epidemics and Research in the Last Forty Years and Prospects for the Future," *American Journal of Tropical Medicine and Hygiene*, Vol. 45, 1991, as cited in Duane J. Gubler, "Emergent and Resurgent Arboviral Diseases As Public Health Problems," in B.W.J. Mahy and D.K. Lvov, eds., *Concepts in Virology: From Ivanovsky to the Present* (Chur, Switzerland: Harwood Academic Publishers, 1993); Vietnam from "World Malaria Situation in 1992: Middle South Asia, Eastern Asia and Oceania," *Weekly Epidemiological Record*, November 4, 1994.

28. WHO member states from Director-General, op. cit. note 3; Odile Frank, Health Situation Analysis and Projection Unit, WHO, Geneva, personal communication, October 6, 1995.

29. Frank, op. cit. note 28.

30. Pinner et al., op. cit. note 20; "tip of the iceberg" from Dr. Marc Lappé, Director, Center for Ethics and Toxic Substances, Gualala, Calif., private communication, March 4, 1996.

31. Pinner et al., op. cit. note 20; Note: There are other sources of undercounting in addition to these. Some diseases result from infections but are not themselves infectious, such as rheumatic heart disease and rheumatoid arthritis. Further complicating matters, some chronic diseases have recently been related to infections, blurring the distinction between the two. Enteroviruses, for example, have been linked to the onset of juvenile diabetes, and *Helicobacter pylori* has turned out to be a major cause of peptic ulcer disease and gastric carcinoma. Some connective tissue diseases are triggered by infections that invade the immune system first, and then spread to other organs and systems. For further discussion see Martin J. Blaser, "The Bacteria Behind Ulcers," *Scientific American*, February 1996.

32. Chrystia Freeland, "Diphtheria Fear in Former USSR," *Financial Times*, June 20, 1995; "Expanded Programme on Immunization: Diphtheria Epidemic in the Newly Independent States of the former USSR, 1990-1994," *Weekly Epidemiological Record*, May 19, 1995.

33. Daniel E. Fountain, Vanga Hospital, Zaire, private communication on ProMED, February 24, 1996 citing Dr. Felix Kuzoe, the WHO Coordinator for Research on African Trypanosomiasis in the Special Program for Research and Training in Tropical Diseases.

34. WHO, op. cit. note 19; world trends from "World Malaria Situation in 1990," WHO, *Weekly Epidemiological Record*, No. 22, 1992; "immense proportions" from Piero Olliaro, Jacqueline Cattani, and Dyann Wirth, "Malaria, the Submerged Disease," *Journal of the American Medical Association*, January 17, 1996; "reporting virtually stopped" from A. Rietveld, WHO, private communication, February 15, 1996.

35. "Tuberculosis Notifications, by WHO Region," *Weekly Epidemiological Record*, March 18, 1994; WHO, Tuberculosis Program, *Tuberculosis Notification Update*, (Geneva: WHO, December 1993); Director-General, "WHO Report on the Tuberculosis Epidemic, 1995: Stop TB at the Source," WHO, Geneva, March 1995.

36. Estimates for 1900 from Biddle, op. cit. note 19.

37. Paul John Dolin, Mario C. Raviglione, and Arata Kochi, *A Review of Current Epidemiological Data and Estimation of Future Tuberculosis Incidence and Mortality* (Geneva: WHO, 1993).

38. Gretchen C. Daily and Paul R. Ehrlich, *Development, Global Change, and The Epidemiological Environment*, Working Paper No. 0062, Stanford University, Morrison Institute for Population and Resources Studies, 1995.

39. Drug-resistant pneumonia from Levy, op. cit. note 4; malaria from David Brown, "When Disease Resists," *Washington Post*, February 14, 1994; HIV data from Director-General, op. cit. note 3; HIV in Asia from John Ward Anderson, "India Seen as Ground Zero in Spread of AIDS to Asia," *Washington Post*, August 17, 1995.

40. J. W. Mason, "The Plague Years," *In These Times*, March 20, 1995; McNeill, op. cit. note 3; Henig, op. cit. note 7.

41. Robert E. Shope, Department of Pathology, University of Texas Medical Branch, Galveston, Texas, private communication, March 5, 1996; Daily and Ehrlich, op. cit. note 38.

42. Lappé, op. cit. note 30.

43. Marc Lappé, *Evolutionary Medicine: Rethinking the Origins of Disease* (San Francisco: Sierra Club Books, 1994).

44. Shope, op. cit. note 41; dead host from Paul Ewald as cited in Weiss, op. cit. note 22.

45. Robert May, "Ecology and Evolution of Host-Virus Associations," in Stephen S. Morse, ed., *Emerging Viruses* (New York: Oxford University Press, 1993); Shope, op. cit. note 41.

46. Mexico from McNeill, op. cit. note 3.

47. Viral traffic from Stephen S. Morse, "Regulating Viral Traffic," *Issues in Science and Technology*, Fall 1990; Morse, op. cit. note 3; Shope, op. cit. note 41.

48. McNeill, op. cit. note 3.

49. Influenza from Christoph Scholtissek, "Cultivating a Killer Virus," *Natural History,* January 1992; Robert G. Webster, "Influenza," in Morse, op. cit., note 45; Associated Press, "Flu Shots for Working-Age People Cut Winter Sick Days, Report Says," *Washington Post,* October 5, 1995; annual cost of influenza from CISET, op. cit. note 2.

50. Air travel from International Air Transport Association (IATA), "Review of Air Transport Development in 1994," in IATA, *World Air Transport Statistics* (Montreal, Que.: 1995); Robert E. Shope and Alfred S. Evans, "Assessing Geographic and Transport Factors, and Recognition of New Viruses," in Morse, op. cit. note 45.

51. Data from Director-General, op. cit. note 3; different mosquitoes from D.J. Gubler and D.W. Trent, "Emergence of Epidemic Dengue/Dengue Hemorrhagic Fever as a Public Health Problem in the Americas," *Infectious Agents and Disease,* Vol. 2, No. 6, 1994.

52. Gubler and Trent, op. cit. note 51.

53. Tire shipment from Lederberg et al., op. cit. note 19; U.S. cities from Robin Marantz Henig, "The New Mosquito Menace," *New York Times,* September 13, 1995; Rajiv Chandrasekaran, "Bold and Bloodthirsty," *Washington Post,* August 17, 1995; Puerto Rico from Jane Stevens, "Dengue Cases on the Rise," *Washington Post,* June 6, 1995.

54. D.J. Gubler, "Dengue and Dengue Hemorrhagic Fever in the Americas," in Southeast Asia Regional Office of WHO, *Dengue/Dengue Hemorrhagic Fever,* Monograph No. 22, New Delhi, 1993.

55. Duane J. Gubler, *Virus Information Exchange Newsletter,* No. 8, 1991 reprinted in Thomas P. Monath, "The Challenge: Biotechnology Transfer to Public Health. Examples from Arbovirology," in David H. Walker, ed., *Global Infectious Diseases: Prevention, Control, and Eradication* (New York: Springer-Verlag, 1992); Morse, op. cit. note 47.

56. James D. Wolfensohn, "1.3 Billion People Living on a Dollar a Day," *Washington Post,* November 13, 1995; Wilken, op. cit. note 10; United Nations, *World Population Prospects: The 1992 Revision* (New York: 1993); studies of health in slums and cities from Trudy Harpham and Carolyn Stephens, "Urbanization and Health in Developing Countries," *World Health Statistics Quarterly,* vol. 44, 1991; for general discussion see Françoise Barten, "Health in a City Environment," *World Health,* May/June 1994; Eugene Linden, "Exploding Cities," *Foreign Affairs Journal,* January/February 1996; Hal Kane, *The Hour of Departure: Forces that Create Refugees and Migrants,* Worldwatch Paper 125 (Washington, D.C.: Worldwatch Institute, June 1995).

57. United Nations Development Program (UNDP), *Human Development Report 1994,* (New York: Oxford University Press, 1994); Nakajima quote from Tacio, op. cit. note 17; Director-General, op. cit. note 3.

58. Associated Press, "Western Health Perils for Poor Nations' Young," *New York Times*, September 24, 1995; Bennett Lorber, "Rattlesnake Powder, Lawn Darts, Hot Tubs, Sushi, and Sex, or Changing Patterns of Infectious Diseases Revisited," *American Journal of Pharmacology*, Vol. 163, 1991.

59. Kinshasa highway from Richard Preston, *The Hot Zone* (New York: Anchor Books/Doubleday, 1994); see also W. Henry Mosley and Peter Cowley, "The Challenge of World Health," *Population Bulletin* (Population Reference Bureau), December 1991.

60. Figure of 11,000 from Jonathan M. Mann and Daniel J.M. Tarantola, "Preventive Medicine: A Broader Approach to the AIDS Crisis," *Harvard International Review*, Fall 1995; "AIDS—Displaying the Global Dynamics," *American Journal of Public Health*, February 1994; Global AIDS data from Aaron Sachs, "HIV/AIDS Cases Rise at Record Rates," in Brown et al. op. cit. note 10; Anderson, op. cit. note 39; Gouri Salvi, "Time Bomb," *Far Eastern Economic Review*, September 21, 1995; John Bongaarts, "Global Trends in AIDS Mortality," *Population and Development Review*, March 1996.

61. Bennett Lorber, Section of Infectious Diseases, Temple University Hospital, Philadelphia, Pennsylvania, private communication, February 26, 1996.

62. Mosley and Cowley, op. cit. note 59; Martin A. Nowak and Andrew J. McMichael, "How HIV Defeats the Immune System," *Scientific American*, August 1995.

63. Lawrence K. Altman, "AIDS is Now the Leading Killer of Americans From 25 to 44," *New York Times*, January 31, 1995; Gina Kolata, "New Picture of Who Will Get AIDS Is Crammed with Addicts," *New York Times*, February 28, 1995.

64. U.S. data from Lappé, op. cit. note 30, and "AIDS Campaign Aimed at Nation's Youth," *The Nation's Health*, January 1996; Uganda data from "Living, and Dying, with the Plague," *The Economist*, February 10, 1996; Philip Shenon, "AIDS Epidemic, Late to Arrive, Now Explodes in Populous Asia," *New York Times*, January 21, 1996; Thailand's current life expectancy from UNDP, *Human Development Report 1995* (New York: UNDP, 1995).

65. Paul Taylor, "AIDS Overwhelming Zimbabwe's Advanced Defenses," *Washington Post*, April 12, 1995; Bongaarts, op. cit. note 60; Director-General, op. cit. note 3.

66. David Brown, "World Bank to Emphasize AIDS as Economic Threat," *Washington Post*, November 28, 1994; $11 billion from Mann and Tarantola, op. cit. note 60; $52 billion from Shenon, op. cit. note 64; Daniel Whelan, "Women, AIDS, and Development," *Peace Review*, Fall 1994.

67. Stephen Buckley, "African AIDS Epidemic Creating a Society of Orphans," *Washington Post*, March 17, 1995; Aaron Sachs, "AIDS Orphans: Africa's Lost Generation," *World Watch*, September\October 1993; *Tanzania: AIDS Assessment and Planning Study*, World Bank Country Study (Washington, D.C.: World Bank, 1992).

68. Monks from Shenon, op. cit. note 64.

69. CARE Australia, "HIV/AIDS in the Countries of the Mekong," *DHA News Special: 1994 in Review* (Geneva: United Nations Department of Humanitarian Affairs, March 1995); STDs from Director-General, op. cit. note 3.

70. McNeill, op. cit. note 3; Biddle, op. cit. note 19.

71. Lappé, op. cit. note 43.

72. Ibid.; Burnet and White, op. cit. note 5; Henig, op. cit. note 7.

73. Manmade malaria from N. L. Karla, *Status Report on Malaria and Other Health-Related Aspects of the Sardar Sarovar Projects, and Recommendations Regarding Short-Term and Long-Term Remedial Measures*, January 1992, as cited in Bradford F. Morse and Thomas R. Berger, *Sardar Sarovar: The Report of the Independent Review* (Ottawa: Resource Futures International Inc., 1992).

74. Rimjhim Jain, "Mosquitoes Storm the Desert," *Down to Earth*, November 30, 1994; Max Martin and Ambika Sharma, "The Microbes Strike Back" *Down to Earth*, January 15, 1995.

75. Ignition wire from Karla, op. cit. note 73.

76. Karl Johnson, "Emerging Viruses in Context: An Overview of Viral Hemorrhagic Fevers," in Morse, op. cit. note 45; 20,000 Argentineans from WHO, "Viral Hemorrhagic Fevers: Report of a WHO Expert Committee," Technical Report No. 712, 1985, as cited in Garrett, op. cit. note 23.

77. Bernard Le Guenno, "Emerging Viruses," *Scientific American*, October 1995; Henig, op. cit. note 7; Garrett, op. cit. note 23.

78. Le Guenno, op. cit. note 77; Johnson, op. cit., note 76.

79. Eliot Marshall, "Hantavirus Outbreak Yields to PCR," *Science*, November 5, 1993; Denise Grady, "Death at the Four Corners," *Discover*, December 1993; Steve Sternberg, "Tracking a Mysterious Killer Virus in the Southwest," *Washington Post*, June 14, 1994.

80. Sternberg, op. cit. note 79.

81. Sternberg, op. cit. note 79; James M. Hughes, C. J. Peters, Mitchell L. Cohen, and Brian W. J. Mahy, "Hantavirus Pulmonary Syndrome: An Emerging Infectious Disease, " *Science*, November 5, 1993; Richard Stone, "The Mouse-Pinon Nut Connection," *Science*, November 5, 1993; Paul R. Epstein, "Emerging Diseases and Ecosystem Instability: New Threats to Public Health," *American Journal of Public Health*, February 1995.

82. Kane, op. cit. note 56; Lappé, op. cit. note 31.

83. Dr. James LeDuc, Division of Communicable Diseases, WHO, Geneva, private communication, March 18, 1996.

84. Japanese encephalitis and general discussion of disruptions from Stephen S. Morse, "Factors in the Emergence of Infectious Diseases," *Emerging Infectious Diseases* (CDC), January/March 1995; LeDuc, op. cit. note 83.

85. Lappé, op. cit. note 43.

86. Richard S. Ostfeld et al., "Ecology of Lyme Disease: Habitat Associations of Ticks *(Ixodes scapularis)* in a Rural Landscape," *Ecological Applications*, Vol. 5, No. 2, 1995; Lappé, op. cit. note 43; Shope, op. cit. note 41.

87. Spread of Lyme disease throughout the U.S. from Lawrence K. Altman, "U.S. Agency Reports Lyme Disease Cases Up by 58% in '94," *New York Times*, June 23, 1995; James E. Herrington, "An Update on Lyme Disease," *Health and Environment Digest*, August 1995; Fishbein and Dennis, op. cit. note 8; Sally Squires, "Warnings Reissued in Wake of Rabies Deaths," *Washington Post*, November 7, 1995; Sue Anne Pressley, "Along the Rio Grande, Waging a Texas-Size War Against Rabies," *Washington Post*, March 8, 1995.

88. Rahul Shrivastava, "A Plague on This Country," *Down to Earth*, October 31, 1994; Meghan Kinney "Plague and Aid," in *Emergency Preparedness News*, Special Edition: "Fighting World Health Crises," October 1994; Paul Epstein, "Climate Change Played a Role in India's Plague," *New York Times*, November 13, 1994.

89. Mahish McDonald, "Surat's Revenge: India Counts the Mounting Costs of Poverty," *Far Eastern Economic Review*, October 13, 1994; Stefan Wagstyl, "A Shock to the System," *Financial Times*, October 5, 1994; John F. Burns, "India's City of Plague: Cesspool of Urban Ills," *New York Times*, October 3, 1994; Laurie Garrett, "The Return of Infectious Disease," *Foreign Affairs*, January/February 1996.

90. Figure of $2 billion from Duane Gubler, CDC, presentation at CISET meeting, Washington, D.C., July 25, 1995; disease surveillance and medical community from Shrivastava, op. cit. note 88; Declan Butler, "India Ponders the Flaws Exposed by Plague," and K. S. Jayaraman and Declan

Butler, "...As Doubts Over Outbreak Rumble On," both in *Nature*, November 10, 1994; Lawrence K. Altman, "Lesson of Plague: Beware of 'Vanquished' Diseases," *New York Times*, September 27, 1994; "Plague: India," *Weekly Epidemiological Record*, February 3, 1995.

91. J. M. Hunter, L. Rey, K. Y.Chu, E. O. Adekolu-John, and K.E. Mott, *Parasitic Diseases in Water Resources Development: The Need for Intersectoral Negotiation* (Geneva: WHO, 1993).

92. J. Almendares, M. Sierra, Pamela K. Anderson, and Paul R. Epstein, "Critical Regions: A Profile of Honduras," *The Lancet*, December 4, 1993.

93. Intergovernmental Panel on Climate Change, Working Group II, Second Assessment Report, "Human Population Health," in *Summary for Policymakers: Impacts, Adaptation and Mitigation Options*, released at a press conference in Washington, D.C., October 24, 1995.

94. M.J. Bouma, H.E. Sondorp, and H.J. van der Kaay, "Climate Change and Periodic Malaria," *The Lancet*, June 4, 1994; Colombia from Paul R. Epstein, Harvard University School of Public Health, Cambridge, Mass., private communication, September 29, 1995; and Will Nixon, "The Heat Is On," *In These Times*, December 11, 1995; RRV from Erwin Jackson, Climate Impacts Unit, Greenpeace International, ProMED communication, citing "River Virus Epidemic Fear," *Sydney Morning Herald*, March 3, 1996; Donald M. Anderson, "Red Tides," *Scientific American*, August 1994.

95. Lack of immunity from Fred Pearce, "Global Alert over Malaria," *New Scientist*, May 13, 1995; Michael E. Loevinsohn, "Climatic Warming and Increased Malaria Incidence in Rwanda," *The Lancet*, March 19, 1994.

96. Encephalitis from Andrew Dobson and Robin Carper, "Biodiversity: Health and Climate Change," *The Lancet*, October 30, 1993; "The Heat Is On," *Down to Earth*, April 30, 1994.

97. Willem J.M. Martens, Jan Rotmans, and Louis W. Niessen, "Climate Change and Malaria Risk: An Integrated Modelling Approach," Global Dynamics and Sustainable Development Program, Research for Man and the Environment (RIVM), National Institute of Public Health and Environmental Protection, The Netherlands, March 1994; Willem J.M. Martens et al., "Potential Risk of Global Climate Change on Malaria Risk," *Environmental Health Perspectives*, May 1995; 60 percent from Robert T. Watson, Associate Director for Environment, Office of Science and Technology Policy, Executive Office of the President, presentation at the American Association for the Advancement of Science meeting, Baltimore, Maryland, February 12, 1996.

98. Martens, Rotmans, and Niessen, op. cit. note 97.

99. W. J. M. Martens, T. H. Jetten, J. Rotmans, and L. W. Niessen, "Climate

Change and Vector-borne Diseases," *Global Environmental Change,* Vol. 5, No. 3, 1995; W. J. M. Martens, "Modelling the Effect of Global Warming on the Prevalence of Schistosomiasis," GLOBO Report No. 10, Global Dynamics and Sustainable Development Program, (RIVM), National Institute of Public Health and Environmental Protection, Maastrict, The Netherlands, July 1995.

100. Morse, op. cit. note 47; Paul R. Epstein, "Climate Forecasting and Health Early Warning Systems," *ProMED Digest,* January 10, 1996.

101. Mark A. Cane, Gidon Eshel, and R. W. Buckland, "Forecasting Zimbabwean Maize Yield Using Eastern Equatorial Pacific Sea Surface Temperature," *Nature,* July 21, 1994; Epstein, Rogers, and Slooff, op. cit. note 16; Morse, op. cit. note 47.

102. "Nearly half" from WHO, *Our Planet, Our Health: Report of the WHO Commission on Health and Environment* (Geneva: WHO, 1992); 80 percent and 25 million deaths from Groupe de Recherche et d'échanges Technologiques (GRET) *Water and Health in Underprivileged Urban Areas* (Paris: Water Solidarity Network, 1994); 10 million deaths per year globally from Linda Nash, "Water Quality and Health," in Peter H. Gleick, ed., *Water in Crisis: A Guide to the World's Fresh Water Resources* (New York: Oxford University Press, 1993).

103. Nash, op. cit. note 102.

104. Director-General, op. cit. note 3; United Nations Children's Emergency Fund (UNICEF), *The State of the World's Children 1995* (New York: Oxford University Press, 1995); 1985 estimates from José Martines, Margaret Phillips, and Richard G. A. Feachem, "Diarrheal Diseases," in Jamison, et al., op. cit. note 23.

105. McNeill, op. cit. note 3; Burnet and White, op. cit. note 5. See also John Snow, *On the Mode of Communication of Cholera,* (London: Oxford University Press, 1936).

106. Carlo Rietveld, the World Bank, "Water Supply and Sanitation in the Context of the Economy in the Developing Countries," paper presented at the Sophia Antipolis Round Table, February 21-23, 1994, as cited in GRET, op. cit. note 102; John Briscoe, "When the Cup Is Half Full: Improving Water and Sanitation Services in the Developing World," *Environment,* May 1993.

107. WHO, *The International Drinking Water Supply and Sanitation Decade: End of Decade Review (as at December 1990);* World Bank, op. cit. note 14.

108. Robert V. Tauxe, Eric D. Mintz, and Robert E. Quick, "Epidemic Cholera in the New World: Translating Field Epidemiology into New Prevention Strategies," *Emerging Infectious Diseases,* October-December

1995; $750 million from Epstein, op. cit. note 94; James Brooke, "How the Cholera Scare is Waking Latin America," *New York Times*, March 8, 1992; "Cholera in 1993, Part I," *Weekly Epidemiological Record*, July 15, 1994; James Brooke, "Cholera Kills 1,100 in Peru and Marches On Reaching the Brazilian Border," *New York Times*, April 19, 1991; Luis Loyola and Patricio Hevia, "Keeping Cholera at Bay," *World Health*, May/June 1993; $200 billion from "The Centers for Disease Control and Prevention Strategy for Emerging Infectious Disease Threats," *Population and Development Review*, September 1994.

109. "Reliably and continuously" from Pan American Health Organization, *Health Conditions in the Americas: Volume I*, Scientific Publication No. 549, (Washington, D.C.: PAHO, 1994); Tauxe, Mintz, and Quick, op. cit. note 108; Denise Barricklow, "Peru's Cholera Conquistadors," *Choices*, April 1992.

110. T. Ramamurthy et al., "Emergence of a Novel Strain of Vibrio Cholerae with Epidemic Potential in Southern and Eastern India," *Lancet,* Vol. 341, 1993, as cited in Tauxe et al., op. cit. note 108; cases from Bradley Sack, International Health Program, Johns Hopkins School of Hygiene and Public Health, private communication, March 1, 1996; Epstein, op. cit. note 81; Martin and Sharma, op. cit. note 74; "Don't Drink the Plankton," *The Economist,* September 23, 1995.

111. Paul R. Epstein, Timothy E. Ford, and Rita R. Colwell, "Marine Ecosystems," *The Lancet,* November 13, 1993; Paul R. Epstein, "Algal Blooms in the Spread and Persistence of Cholera," *BioSystems*, Vol. 31, 1993.

112. Ruby Ofori, "Dam Brings a Bitter Harvest," Inter Press Service, in TDR, op. cit. note 19; Hermann Feldmeier, "Sugar Cane and Bilharziasis in the Sahel," *Swiss Review of World Affairs*, November 1995.

113. Ibid.

114. Hunter, et al., op. cit. note 91.

115. Ofori, op. cit. note 112.

116. McNeill, op. cit. note 3.

117. Director-General, op. cit. note 3.

118. WHO Expert Committee on Onchocerciasis Control, *Onchocerciasis and Its Control*, WHO Technical Report No. 852 (Geneva: WHO, 1995); James A. Lee, "Health Considerations for Economic Development," in *The Environment, Public Health and Human Ecology: Considerations for Economic Development,* (Baltimore, Maryland: World Bank/Johns Hopkins University Press, 1985).

119. World Bank, op. cit. note 14.

120. The World Bank, *World Development Report 1992* (Washington, D.C., 1992).

121. Philip Wan, "Clean Water and Environment: Women and Children at Particular Risk," *Waterfront: Water Supply, Environmental Sanitation and Hygiene News* (New York: UNICEF, December 1994).

122. 1.7 billion and 12 percent from WHO, op. cit. note 107; 60 percent from World Bank, op. cit. note 120; solar cooker from Christopher Flavin and Nicholas Lenssen, *Power Surge: Guide to the Coming Energy Revolution* (New York: W.W. Norton, 1994).

123. UNEP Regional Office for Europe, "Bad Water Kills 25,000 People a Day," *DHA News Special: 1994 in Review,* No. 13 (Geneva: United Nations Department of Humanitarian Affairs (DHA), March 1995); László Somlyódy, "Managing Water Quality in Central and Eastern Europe," *Options,* Summer 1994.

124. The figure 75 percent from Angela Charlton, "Study By Russia Calls Its Ecology a Nightmare," *Journal of Commerce,* February 6, 1995; Chrystia Freeland, "Virulent Symptoms of Social Decay," *Financial Times,* June 17-18, 1995; 128 and 300 percent figures from Michael Specter, "Russia's Declining Health: Rising Illness, Shorter Lives," *New York Times,* February 19, 1995; Black Sea from Michael Specter, "Russia Moves on Cholera Epidemic in South," *New York Times,* August 20, 1994; Andrei Ivanov and Judith Perera, "Another Cholera Outbreak in Ukraine; Russia on Alert," InterPress Service, July 4, 1995; plankton detection from Epstein, op. cit. note 94.

125. Robert D. Morris and Ronnie Levin, "Estimating the Incidence of Waterborne Infectious Disease Related to Drinking Water in the United States," in Eric G. Reichard and Giovanni A. Zapponi, eds., *Assessing and Managing Health Risks from Drinking Water Contamination: Approaches and Applications* (Proceedings of a symposium organized by the National Water Research Institute, the International Commission on Groundwater, and the Istituto Superiore di Sanita, held in Rome, September 1994), International Association of Hydrological Sciences, Velp, the Netherlands, IAHS Publication No. 233, 1995; U.S. data and cryptosporidious at low dose from Gunther F. Craun, "Waterborne Disease Outbreaks in the United States of America: Causes and Prevention," *World Health Statistics Quarterly,* Vol. 45, 1992.

126. The 40 percent figure from "The Health Costs of Drinking Water Contamination: Waterborne Infectious Disease," *Environmental and Energy Study Institute Weekly Bulletin,* Washington, D.C., August 15, 1994; England and The Netherlands from Stephen S. Morse, Rockefeller University, New York City, private communication, September 29, 1995; North America from Pierre Payment et al., "A Randomized Trial to Evaluate the Risk of

Gastrointestinal Disease due to Consumption of Drinking Water Meeting Current Microbiological Standards," *American Journal of Public Health*, June 1991.

127. Ronnie Levin and Winston Harrington, "Infectious Waterborne Disease and Disinfection By-Products in the US: Costs of Disease," *Abstracts: Regulatory Issues* in Reichard and Zapponi, op. cit. note 125.

128. "Rescue Attempt for the Guarapiranga Water Basin," *Water Newsletter: Developments in Water, Sanitation, and Environment* (International Water and Sanitation Center, The Hague), July 1994.

129. "Guinea Worm: Disease-free Countries to be Certified," *Water Newsletter: Developments in Water, Sanitation and Environment,* (International Water and Sanitation Center, The Hague), September 1995, based on "Guinea Worm: Countries to be Certified Cleared," *TDR News,* November 1994.

130. "The End of the Worm is Nigh," *The Economist,* December 2, 1995; John Schwartz, "Worm Disease Nearing Extinction," *Washington Post,* December 5, 1995; "Decline of Dracunculiasis Cases, 1987-1993," *Weekly Epidemiological Record*, April 27, 1994.

131. ORT data from UNICEF, op. cit. note 104; Director-General, op. cit. note 3.

132. Biddle, op. cit. note 36; David McCullough, *The Path Between the Seas: the Creation of the Panama Canal, 1870-1914* (New York: Simon and Schuster, 1977).

133. David Brown, "'Wonder Drugs' Losing Healing Aura," *Washington Post*, June 26, 1995; Brown, op. cit. note 39.

134. Levy, op. cit. note 4.

135. Fleming quote in Levy, op. cit. note 4, citing *New York Times,* June 26, 1945.

136. Smith, op. cit. note 5.

137. Levy quote from presentation at the Institute of Medicine, 25th Anniversary Meeting, National Academy of Sciences, Washington, D.C., October 16, 1995; Brown, op. cit. note 133.

138. American Society of Microbiology, *Report of the ASM Task Force on Antibiotic Resistance* (Washington, D.C.: 1995); Tim Beardsley, "Resisting Resistance," *Scientific American,* January 1996; $9 billion from "Health—the Facts," *New Internationalist,* October 1995 as cited in G. Cannon, *Superbug: Nature's Revenge* (London: Virgin Books, 1995).

139. Half from Institute of Medicine, *Human Health Risks with the Subtherapeutic Use of Penicillin or Tetracyclines in Animal Feed*, National Academy Press, Washington, D.C., 1989) as cited in ASM, op. cit. note 138.

140. Dr. Stuart Levy, personal communication, June 6, 1995; see Levy, op. cit. note 4, for more discussion on antibiotics in agricultural settings.

141. Levy, op. cit. note 4; New Guinea from ASM, op. cit. note 138; Sharon Kingman, "Resistance a European Problem, Too," *Science*, April 15, 1994; Atlanta from Jo Hofman et al., "The Prevalence of Drug-Resistant *Streptococcus pneumoniae* in Atlanta," *New England Journal of Medicine*, August 24, 1995.

142. ASM, op. cit. note 138; Bernice Wuethrich, "Migrating Genes Could Spread Resistance," *New Scientist*, October 15, 1994; Levy, op. cit. note 4; Brown, op. cit. note 133; NCID, op. cit. note 12.

143. Gene Bylinsky, "The New Fight Against Killer Microbes," *Fortune*, September 5, 1994; Levy, op. cit. note 4; $4 billion from ASM, op. cit. note 138; U.S. Congress Office of Technology Assessment, *Impacts of Antibiotic-Resistant Bacteria*, OTA-H-629 (Washington, D.C.: Government Printing Office, September 1995); $100 to $200 million from Ann Gibbons, "Exploring New Strategies to Fight Drug-resistant Microbes," *Science*, Vol. 257, 1992, as cited in Lappé, op. cit. note 43.

144. Iceland from Joan Stephenson, "Icelandic Researchers Are Showing the Way to Bring Down Rates of Antibiotic-Resistant Bacteria," *Journal of the American Medical Association*, January 17, 1996.

145. "CDC Backs More Sparing Use of Antibiotics," *Washington Post*, September 29, 1995; for more recommendations see NCID, op. cit. note 12; Lederberg, Shope, and Oaks, op. cit., note 53; Brown, op. cit., note 133.

146. Burnet and White, op. cit. note 5; Robert Chen, Lynelle Phillips, and Steve Hadler, "Bottom Line: Vaccination Benefits Far Outweigh Risks," *The Nation's Health*, December, 1995.

147. Hal Kane, "Immunization Rates Soar," in Lester R. Brown, Hal Kane, and David Malin Roodman, *Vital Signs 1994* (New York: W.W. Norton, 1994); Foster et al., op. cit. note 23; Samuel L. Katz and Bruce G. Gellin, "Measles Vaccine: Do We Need New Vaccines or New Programs?" *Science*, September 2, 1994.

148. C. Everett Koop, "In the Dark About Shots," *Washington Post*, February 10, 1993.

149. Associated Press, "U.S. Trails Poor Nations in Early Innoculation," *Washington Post*, June 6, 1993; Associated Press, "Million Toddlers Said to Need Vaccinations," *Washington Post*, May 5, 1995.

150. McDonald's from "Time to Immunize!" *Washington Post,* August 29, 1995; Laura Petrecca, "A Shot at Good Health for Inner-City Kids," *USA Today,* January 10, 1996.

151. Peter Aldhous, "Vaccine Shows Promise in Tanzania Test," *Science,* November 4, 1994; Phyllida Brown, "Two Cheers for a New Vaccine," *World Press Review,* February 1995, based on her article in *New Scientist,* November 5, 1994.

152. Lester R. Brown et al., *State of the World 1996* (New York: W.W. Norton, 1996); Lester R. Brown, Christopher Flavin, and Sandra Postel, *Saving the Planet: How to Shape and Envrionmentally Sustainable Global Economy* (New York: W.W. Norton, 1991); Lester R. Brown and Hal Kane, *Full House: Reassessing the Earth's Population Carrying Capacity* (New York: W.W. Norton, 1994); Sandra Postel, *Last Oasis: Facing Water Scarcity* (New York: W.W. Norton, 1992); Flavin and Lenssen, op. cit. note 122.

153. Donatus de Silva, "Vaccinating Against War," *Our Planet,* Vol. 7, No. 3, 1995.

154. Oyewale Tomori, College of Medicine, Ibadan, Nigeria, private communication to Stephen S. Morse, Rockefeller University, October 30, 1993; John Mugabe, "Africa Must Raise its Budgets for Human Health Research," *Biotechnology and Development Monitor,* December 1993; D.A. Henderson, "Strategies for the Twenty-First Century: Control or Eradication?" *Archives of Virology,* Special Issue: 1992.

155. Forty-Eighth World Health Assembly, "Communicable Diseases Prevention and Control: New, Emerging, and Re-emerging Infectious Diseases," (Geneva, WHO, May 12, 1995).

156. T. Demetri Vacalis, Christopher L.R. Bartlett, and Cheryl G. Shapiro, "Electronic Communication and the Future of International Public Health Surveillance," *Emerging Infectious Diseases,* January/March 1995; Dorothy Preslar, Washington ProMED Officer, Federation of American Scientists, private communication, July 14, 1995; Ebola from John Schwartz, "Computers Used to Fight A Much Deadlier Virus," *Washington Post,* May 20, 1995; Ebola and computer users from John Woodall, ProMED List Moderator, New York State Department of Health, Albany, N.Y., "Moderator's Account: The Ebola Outbreak," May 8, 1995.

157. Epstein, Rogers, and Slooff, op. cit. note 16.

PUBLICATION ORDER FORM

No. of
Copies

_____ 61. **Electricity's Future: The Shift to Efficiency and Small-Scale Power**
        by Christopher Flavin.
_____ 63. **Energy Productivity: Key to Environmental Protection and Economic Progress**
        by William U. Chandler.
_____ 65. **Reversing Africa's Decline** by Lester R. Brown and Edward C. Wolf.
_____ 66. **World Oil: Coping With the Dangers of Success** by Christopher Flavin.
_____ 68. **Banishing Tobacco** by William U. Chandler.
_____ 70. **Electricity For A Developing World: New Directions** by Christopher Flavin.
_____ 75. **Reassessing Nuclear Power: The Fallout From Chernobyl** by Christopher Flavin.
_____ 77. **The Future of Urbanization: Facing the Ecological and Economic Constraints**
        by Lester R. Brown and Jodi L. Jacobson.
_____ 78. **On the Brink of Extinction: Conserving The Diversity of Life** by Edward C. Wolf.
_____ 79. **Defusing the Toxics Threat: Controlling Pesticides and Industrial Waste**
        by Sandra Postel.
_____ 80. **Planning the Global Family** by Jodi L. Jacobson.
_____ 81. **Renewable Energy: Today's Contribution, Tomorrow's Promise** by
        Cynthia Pollock Shea.
_____ 82. **Building on Success: The Age of Energy Efficiency** by Christopher Flavin
        and Alan B. Durning.
_____ 84. **Rethinking the Role of the Automobile** by Michael Renner.
_____ 86. **Environmental Refugees: A Yardstick of Habitability** by Jodi L. Jacobson.
_____ 89. **National Security: The Economic and Environmental Dimensions** by Michael Renner.
_____ 90. **The Bicycle: Vehicle for a Small Planet** by Marcia D. Lowe.
_____ 91. **Slowing Global Warming: A Worldwide Strategy** by Christopher Flavin
_____ 92. **Poverty and the Environment: Reversing the Downward Spiral** by Alan B. Durning.
_____ 93. **Water for Agriculture: Facing the Limits** by Sandra Postel.
_____ 94. **Clearing the Air: A Global Agenda** by Hilary F. French.
_____ 95. **Apartheid's Environmental Toll** by Alan B. Durning.
_____ 96. **Swords Into Plowshares: Converting to a Peace Economy** by Michael Renner.
_____ 97. **The Global Politics of Abortion** by Jodi L. Jacobson.
_____ 98. **Alternatives to the Automobile: Transport for Livable Cities** by Marcia D. Lowe.
_____ 99. **Green Revolutions: Environmental Reconstruction in Eastern Europe and the**
        Soviet Union by Hilary F. French.
_____100. **Beyond the Petroleum Age: Designing a Solar Economy** by Christopher Flavin
        and Nicholas Lenssen.
_____101. **Discarding the Throwaway Society** by John E. Young.
_____102. **Women's Reproductive Health: The Silent Emergency** by Jodi L. Jacobson.
_____103. **Taking Stock: Animal Farming and the Environment** by Alan B. Durning and
        Holly B. Brough.
_____104. **Jobs in a Sustainable Economy** by Michael Renner.
_____105. **Shaping Cities: The Environmental and Human Dimensions** by Marcia D. Lowe.
_____106. **Nuclear Waste: The Problem That Won't Go Away** by Nicholas Lenssen.
_____107. **After the Earth Summit: The Future of Environmental Governance**
        by Hilary F. French.
_____108. **Life Support: Conserving Biological Diversity** by John C. Ryan.
_____109. **Mining the Earth** by John E. Young.
_____110. **Gender Bias: Roadblock to Sustainable Development** by Jodi L. Jacobson.
_____111. **Empowering Development: The New Energy Equation** by Nicholas Lenssen.
_____112. **Guardians of the Land: Indigenous Peoples and the Health of the Earth**
        by Alan Thein Durning.
_____113. **Costly Tradeoffs: Reconciling Trade and the Environment** by Hilary F. French.
_____114. **Critical Juncture: The Future of Peacekeeping** by Michael Renner.
_____115. **Global Network: Computers in a Sustainable Society** by John E. Young.
_____116. **Abandoned Seas: Reversing the Decline of the Oceans** by Peter Weber.
_____117. **Saving the Forests: What Will It Take?** by Alan Thein Durning.

_____ **Total Copies**

Single Copy: $5.00   •   2–5: $4.00 ea.   •   6–20: $3.00 ea. •   21 or more: $2.00 ea.
Call Director of Communication at (202) 452-1999 to inquire about discounts on larger orders.

☐ **Membership in the Worldwatch Library: $30.00 (international airmail $45.00)**
The paperback edition of our 250-page "annual physical of the planet,"
State of the World, plus all Worldwatch Papers released during the calendar year.

☐ **Subscription to *World Watch* magazine: $20.00 (international airmail $35.00)**
Stay abreast of global environmental trends and issues with our award-winning,
eminently readable bimonthly magazine.

☐ **Worldwatch Database Disk Subscription: One year for $89**
Includes current global agricultural, energy, economic, environmental, social, and
military indicators from all current Worldwatch publications. Includes a mid-year
update, and *Vital Signs* and *State of the World* as they are published. Can be used
with Lotus 1-2-3, Quattro Pro, Excel, SuperCalc and many other spreadsheets.
Check one: _____high-density IBM-compatible or   _____Macintosh

---

Make check payable to Worldwatch Institute
1776 Massachusetts Avenue, N.W., Washington, D.C. 20036-1904 USA

Please include $3 postage and handling for non-subscription orders.

Enclosed is my check for U.S. $_____
AMEX ☐ VISA ☐ Mastercard ☐ _____

Card Number   Expiration Date

---

name   **daytime phone #**

---

address

---

city   **state   zip/country**

Phone: (202) 452-1999   Fax: (202) 296-7365   E-Mail: wwpub@igc.apc.org   WWP

PUBLICATION ORDER FORM

No. of
Copies

_____ 61. **Electricity's Future: The Shift to Efficiency and Small-Scale Power**
by Christopher Flavin.
_____ 63. **Energy Productivity: Key to Environmental Protection and Economic Progress**
by William U. Chandler.
_____ 65. **Reversing Africa's Decline** by Lester R. Brown and Edward C. Wolf.
_____ 66. **World Oil: Coping With the Dangers of Success** by Christopher Flavin.
_____ 68. **Banishing Tobacco** by William U. Chandler.
_____ 70. **Electricity For A Developing World: New Directions** by Christopher Flavin.
_____ 75. **Reassessing Nuclear Power: The Fallout From Chernobyl** by Christopher Flavin.
_____ 77. **The Future of Urbanization: Facing the Ecological and Economic Constraints**
by Lester R. Brown and Jodi L. Jacobson.
_____ 78. **On the Brink of Extinction: Conserving The Diversity of Life** by Edward C. Wolf.
_____ 79. **Defusing the Toxics Threat: Controlling Pesticides and Industrial Waste**
by Sandra Postel.
_____ 80. **Planning the Global Family** by Jodi L. Jacobson.
_____ 81. **Renewable Energy: Today's Contribution, Tomorrow's Promise** by
Cynthia Pollock Shea.
_____ 82. **Building on Success: The Age of Energy Efficiency** by Christopher Flavin
and Alan B. Durning.
_____ 84. **Rethinking the Role of the Automobile** by Michael Renner.
_____ 86. **Environmental Refugees: A Yardstick of Habitability** by Jodi L. Jacobson.
_____ 89. **National Security: The Economic and Environmental Dimensions** by Michael Renner.
_____ 90. **The Bicycle: Vehicle for a Small Planet** by Marcia D. Lowe.
_____ 91. **Slowing Global Warming: A Worldwide Strategy** by Christopher Flavin
_____ 92. **Poverty and the Environment: Reversing the Downward Spiral** by Alan B. Durning.
_____ 93. **Water for Agriculture: Facing the Limits** by Sandra Postel.
_____ 94. **Clearing the Air: A Global Agenda** by Hilary F. French.
_____ 95. **Apartheid's Environmental Toll** by Alan B. Durning.
_____ 96. **Swords Into Plowshares: Converting to a Peace Economy** by Michael Renner.
_____ 97. **The Global Politics of Abortion** by Jodi L. Jacobson.
_____ 98. **Alternatives to the Automobile: Transport for Livable Cities** by Marcia D. Lowe.
_____ 99. **Green Revolutions: Environmental Reconstruction in Eastern Europe and the
Soviet Union** by Hilary F. French.
_____100. **Beyond the Petroleum Age: Designing a Solar Economy** by Christopher Flavin
and Nicholas Lenssen.
_____101. **Discarding the Throwaway Society** by John E. Young.
_____102. **Women's Reproductive Health: The Silent Emergency** by Jodi L. Jacobson.
_____103. **Taking Stock: Animal Farming and the Environment** by Alan B. Durning and
Holly B. Brough.
_____104. **Jobs in a Sustainable Economy** by Michael Renner.
_____105. **Shaping Cities: The Environmental and Human Dimensions** by Marcia D. Lowe.
_____106. **Nuclear Waste: The Problem That Won't Go Away** by Nicholas Lenssen.
_____107. **After the Earth Summit: The Future of Environmental Governance**
by Hilary F. French.
_____108. **Life Support: Conserving Biological Diversity** by John C. Ryan.
_____109. **Mining the Earth** by John E. Young.
_____110. **Gender Bias: Roadblock to Sustainable Development** by Jodi L. Jacobson.
_____111. **Empowering Development: The New Energy Equation** by Nicholas Lenssen.
_____112. **Guardians of the Land: Indigenous Peoples and the Health of the Earth**
by Alan Thein Durning.
_____113. **Costly Tradeoffs: Reconciling Trade and the Environment** by Hilary F. French.
_____114. **Critical Juncture: The Future of Peacekeeping** by Michael Renner.
_____115. **Global Network: Computers in a Sustainable Society** by John E. Young.
_____116. **Abandoned Seas: Reversing the Decline of the Oceans** by Peter Weber.
_____117. **Saving the Forests: What Will It Take?** by Alan Thein Durning.

_____ **Total Copies**

Single Copy: $5.00 • 2–5: $4.00 ea. • 6–20: $3.00 ea. • 21 or more: $2.00 ea.
Call Director of Communication at (202) 452-1999 to inquire about discounts on larger orders.

☐ **Membership in the Worldwatch Library: $30.00 (international airmail $45.00)**
The paperback edition of our 250-page "annual physical of the planet,"
State of the World, plus all Worldwatch Papers released during the calendar year.

☐ **Subscription to *World Watch* magazine: $20.00 (international airmail $35.00)**
Stay abreast of global environmental trends and issues with our award-winning, eminently readable bimonthly magazine.

☐ **Worldwatch Database Disk Subscription: One year for $89**
Includes current global agricultural, energy, economic, environmental, social, and military indicators from all current Worldwatch publications. Includes a mid-year update, and *Vital Signs* and *State of the World* as they are published. Can be used with Lotus 1-2-3, Quattro Pro, Excel, SuperCalc and many other spreadsheets.
Check one: _____high-density IBM-compatible or _____Macintosh

Make check payable to Worldwatch Institute
1776 Massachusetts Avenue, N.W., Washington, D.C. 20036-1904 USA

Please include $3 postage and handling for non-subscription orders.

Enclosed is my check for U.S. $_____
AMEX☐ VISA☐ Mastercard☐ _____
                                Card Number   Expiration Date

name   **daytime phone #**

address

city   **state**   **zip/country**
Phone: (202) 452-1999   Fax: (202) 296-7365   E-Mail: wwpub@igc.apc.org   WWP